TOM'S
DAILY PLAN

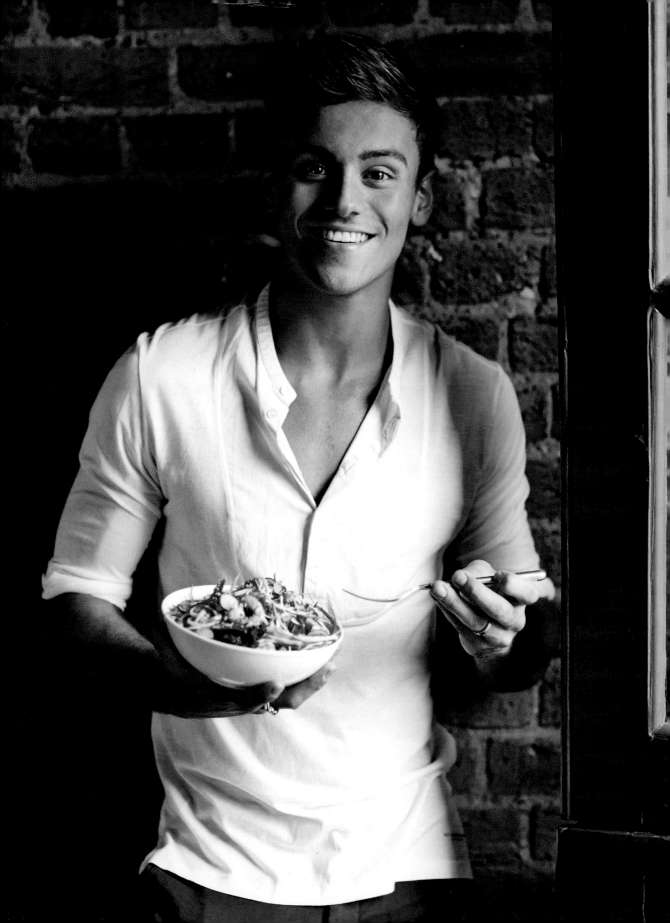

TOM'S
DAILY PLAN

TOM DALEY

I dedicate this book to my dad, Rob.
It was always my mission in life to get him to exercise,
and although he succeeded in getting me to eat my veggies,
I never quite managed to get him to fall in love with exercise.
But maybe if he saw this book, he would give it a go.

HQ, an imprint of HarperCollins*Publishers*, 1 London Bridge Street, London, SE1 9GF

www.harpercollins.co.uk

First published by HQ, an imprint of HarperCollins*Publishers* 2016

Text © Tom Daley 2016

10 9 8 7 6 5 4 3 2 1

Tom Daley asserts the moral right to be identified as the author of this work

A catalogue record of this book is available from the British Library

Paperback edition ISBN 978-0-00-821229-2
Signed edition ISBN 978-0-00-821231-5

Design: Smith & Gilmour
Editor: Jinny Johnson
Photography: Dan Jones
Food stylist: Emily Jonzen
Props stylist: Morag Farquhar
Clothes stylist: Emily Giffard-Taylor
Clothes: Adidas, J Crew, Oliver Sweeney, Club Monaco, J Lindeberg, ASOS
Make-up: Victoria Penrose
Nutritionist: Fiona Hunter, BSc (Hons) Nutrition, Dip Dietectics

Printed and bound in Italy

≈ CONTENTS ≈

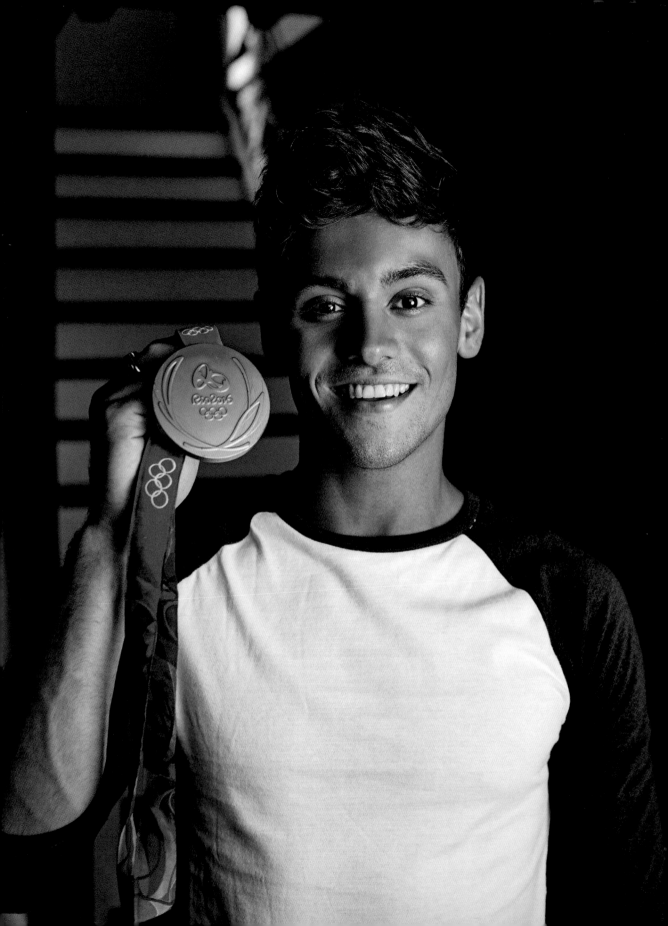

~ WELCOME TO ~ MY DAILY PLAN

As an Olympian, it's my job to know all about eating healthily as well as getting – and staying! – fit. I have learned a huge amount about food and nutrition and I've spent a lot of time trying to learn about my body so I can perform to the best of my ability. But I've also worked with a lot of experts on lifestyle factors, such as willpower, motivation, achieving a healthy work/life balance, and it's amazing how much of a difference that can really make. I wanted to write this book so I could share some of these ideas, because I know they will work for you too.

My plan will show you how to eat well, build strength, tone up and train both your body and mind to reach your health and fitness goals in easy, accessible steps. The following pages feature more than 80 of my favourite recipes for quick, delicious and easy-to-prepare meals, home workouts for all fitness levels, and lifestyle tips to improve your overall performance. My aim is to help you achieve your best and feel amazing, all day, every day.

What's the plan? It's simple, and I promise you don't have to follow my Olympic training schedule of five hours, six days a week!

• EAT All my recipes are truly delicious. Mix and match the breakfasts, lunches and dinners that will work for your day, and don't be scared to add in a treat too.

• MOVE Follow my customised fitness routines five days a week. These are QUICK and it doesn't matter how fit – or not – you are. Just 20 minutes a day will really help.

• LIVE Make some 'you time' with my daily life hacks. They are designed to keep you firmly on track with your new healthy, happier lifestyle.

YOU ARE WHAT YOU EAT

We all lead busy lives and it's all too easy to fall into a pattern of grabbing unhealthy food on the go or trying the latest fad diets. These diets do not work and they go against the basic principles of nutrition and the way your body functions.

I love food and my food memories all involve great meals with my family. My mum always cooked for us when we were growing up and Sunday roast dinners were a real ritual with all the family, including my grandparents, sitting around the table talking and laughing.

I think making food a social occasion is really important, so rather than eating at your desk or in front of the TV, sit down at the table and create your own food rituals.

MY AIM IS TO HELP YOU BE YOUR BEST AND FEEL AMAZING, ALL DAY, EVERY DAY

I enjoy cooking and experimenting with new dishes and food is an important part of my social life; I often make dinner for my friends, and my fiancé Lance and I always take time out to cook and eat a meal together.

MY RECIPES

The recipes in this book will give you a balance of nutritious foods, meaning you will never be hungry – and they are so tasty, you'll want to cook them time and time again. Most are easy to prepare – you're not going to spend hours and hours in the kitchen chopping and stirring. I don't have time for that either!

All my recipes can be cooked on a budget; you'll be able to buy the ingredients at your local shop or you'll already have many of them your store cupboard. I promise you won't have to hunt down lots of strange-sounding items!

For me, breakfast is the most important meal of the day so I've included all my favourite breakfast recipes and hope you enjoy them too. Then there are plenty of soups and salads, delicious supper dishes and some weekend specials – even my mum's Sunday roast! – for days when you might have a little more time in the kitchen.

By the way, I do love chilli and I add it to quite a lot of dishes. If you're not a fan, just leave it out!

We all need to cut down on sugar and the less you eat, the less you will crave, but I had to feature a few treats! Most are sweetened with honey or maple syrup or using the natural sweetness of fruit. I never deny myself and think that it's important to allow yourself the occasional treat.

Having regular snacks will ensure you're always energised. I like a snack right after training. While your body can store fat and carbohydrates, it does not store protein, so it has no reservoir to draw from when you are running low. After training is when muscle is sensitive to nutrients that it can use to repair and grow. Try the protein shakes or the power balls in the snacks chapter in this book – they are delicious!

CALORIES IN, CALORIES OUT

For many people, losing weight and looking good is simplified into the equation of calories in versus calories out – if you use up more calories through exercise than you eat, you will lose weight. In fact, it's more complex than this and in order to fuel your mind and body properly, you should never deprive yourself of any food groups or deliberately go hungry.

The recipes in this book are not intended to be a calorie-counted regime, but they are well balanced and do not include empty calories in the form of refined carbs, or lots of salt or sugar. There is a calorie count for each one, should you want to know, plus there are full nutritional details for the recipes at the back of the book.

GET MOVING

Every person is unique and you will have individual energy demands, according to your age, weight, activity levels and so on. Whether you have a very active job, are on your feet all day running around after children, or you sit at a desk most of the time, it's important to listen to your body and to eat foods that make you feel energised, nourished and strong, so you achieve the results you want.

My Daily Workouts are designed for time-poor people and require no extra equipment outside of what you already have at home. I've designed 20-minute routines that can be adapted, depending on your ability, for five days of the week, with two rest days.

Alongside these workouts, the more exercise and activity you can build into your everyday life, the better. So whether it's taking the stairs, cycling to work, dancing around the house or using the latest apps and technology to track your activity, every small change helps.

BOOST YOUR BRAIN

What you eat and drink is not only fuel for your body but also fuel for your brain. After the Olympic Games in 2012, I went through a phase of not eating as well as I should – I was going out a lot and drinking too much. Soon I found that I wasn't performing well in the diving pool and I had no energy; my mood was low and I found myself caught up in negative thinking patterns. I knew there was no quick fix. I had to get back to focusing on what I was eating and making other changes, so I could start performing well again.

Stress and tiredness make us crave unhealthy and sugary foods and it's so easy to get stuck on what I call 'the sugar train' – starting the day with unhealthy sugar-packed cereal, which sets you on a cycle of blood sugar spike and then crash.

The way we think and feel are central to the food and lifestyle choices we make. With mental strength in mind, I have included some lifestyle tips in the book to help you eliminate stress, change negative thought patterns, improve energy levels and effectively manage your time and reach your goals. There are also tips about the importance of sleep, secrets to increase your exercise performance, and a simple meditation routine to help you feel calm, centred and happy.

PLAN, PREPARE, PERFORM!

In my world, where physical and mental strength are of the greatest importance, this is one of the mottos that I live by. And I believe that planning your meals, your exercise and your rest and relaxation is vital for everyone's health and happiness. You may not be able to follow your plan to the letter, but it's a great start and will help you feel good from the inside out.

Eat well, exercise with enthusiasm and calm your mind – and you'll soon start to look and feel amazing!

GOOD LUCK!

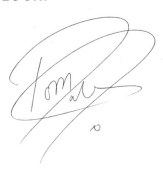

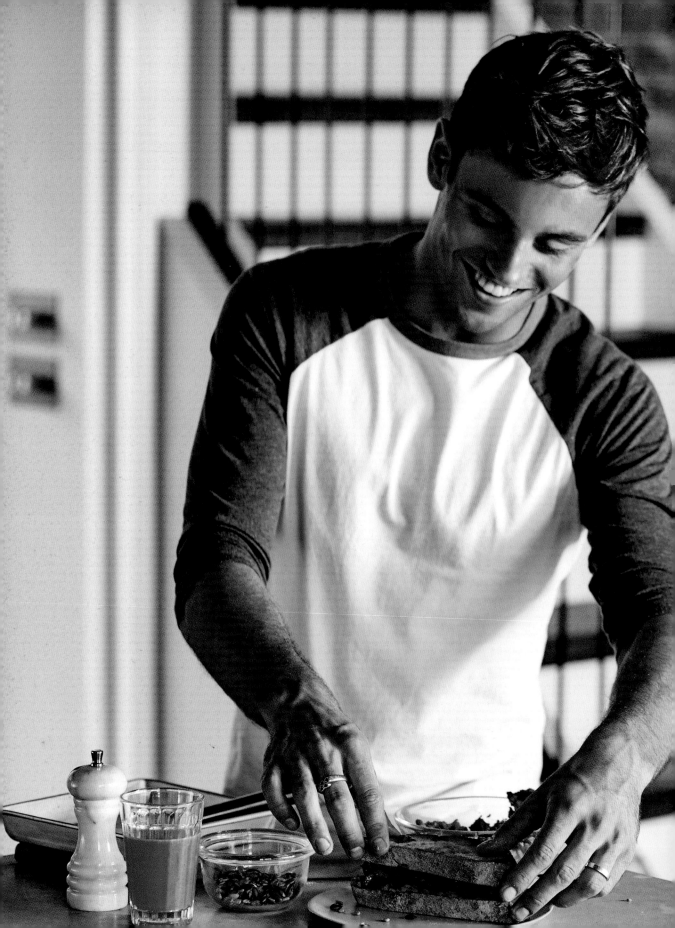

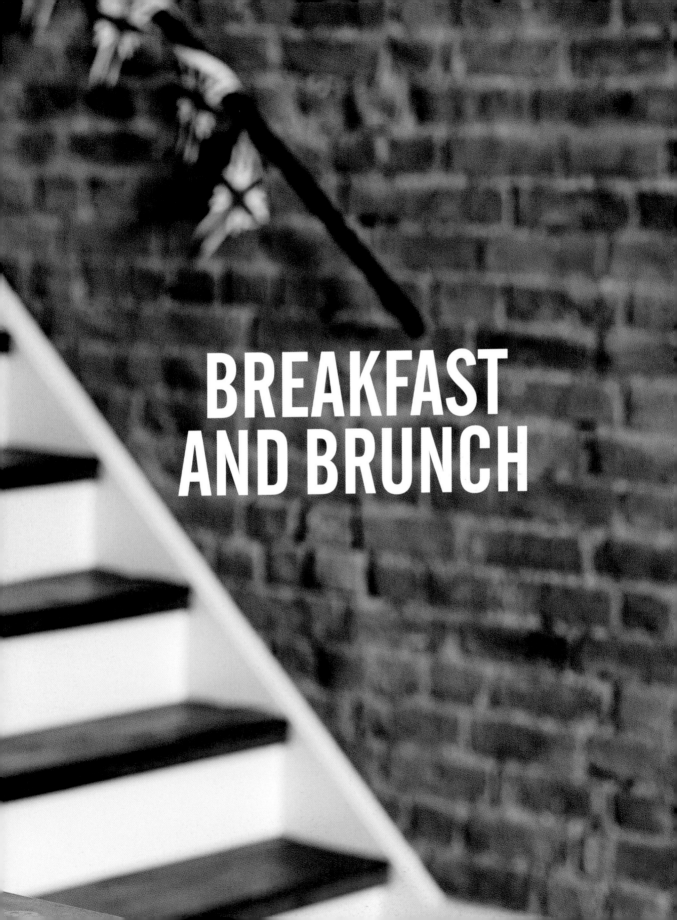

BREAKFAST AND BRUNCH

≈ PLUM YOGHURT POTS ≈

If you're a get-up-and-go person, like me, this is an ideal breakfast that you can prepare the night before so it's ready to enjoy at home or to take to work with you. This recipe tastes good with plums or see my other ideas for using other fruits, such as bananas or strawberries, below.

SERVES 2

265 CALORIES PER SERVING

2 large plums, chopped

½ tsp maple syrup

½ tsp ground mixed spice

juice of ½ orange

200g full-fat Greek yoghurt

50ml whole milk

20g oat bran

15g flaked almonds, toasted

1 Put the plums in a bowl and toss them with the maple syrup, mixed spice and orange juice.

2 Mix the yoghurt, milk and oat bran together and spoon this mixture into 2 x 300ml pots. You can use glass tumblers or plastic sealable pots – whatever you prefer.

3 Add the plums, scatter the flaked almonds on top and cover the pots with cling film or lids until you're ready to eat.

VARIATIONS

BANANA YOGHURT POTS

324 CALORIES PER SERVING

Slice a large banana and divide the slices between the pots. Prepare the yoghurt mixture as above, then pile it into the pots and sprinkle with a pinch of cinnamon. Toast 8 pecan nuts in a dry frying pan, then chop them and scatter them over each pot.

STRAWBERRY YOGHURT POTS

221 CALORIES PER SERVING

Roughly chop 100g of strawberries and toss them with the juice of half an orange, half a teaspoon of balsamic vinegar and half a teaspoon of honey. Divide the fruit between the pots. Top with the yoghurt mixture, then scatter 15g of chopped pistachios on top.

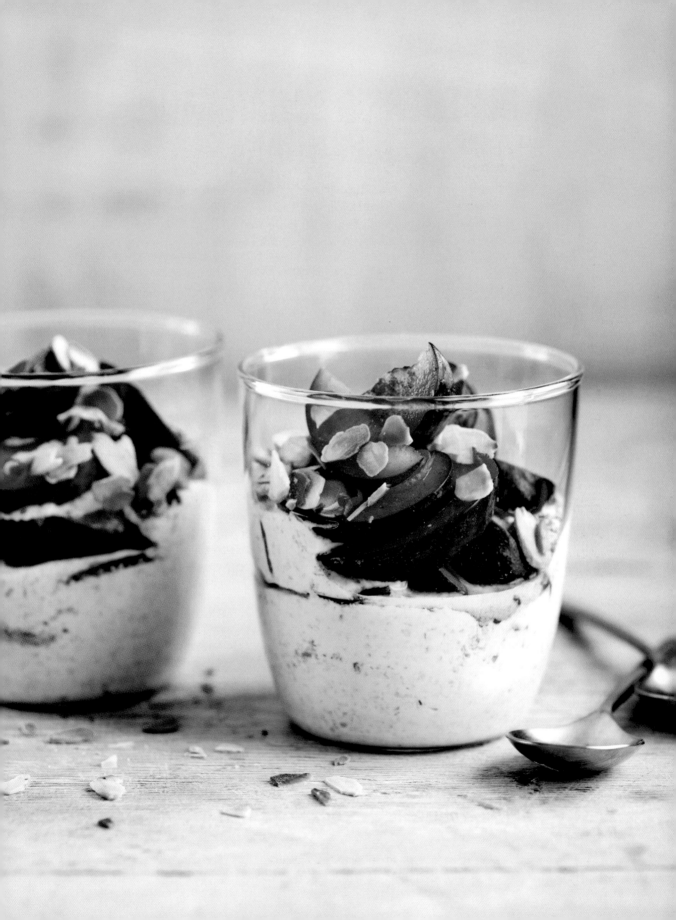

~ BLUEBERRY, BANANA AND ~ SEED PANCAKES

Who doesn't love pancakes? This is a change from the traditional recipe and it's packed with fibre and vitamins. It satisfies my sweet tooth too! The seeds and oat bran will help to fill you up or you can add some protein powder for a post workout boost.

SERVES 2

97 CALORIES PER PANCAKE

1 banana, chopped

1 medium egg

100ml whole milk

2 tbsp oat bran or protein powder

pinch of cinnamon

100g blueberries

1 tsp chia seeds or linseeds

1 tsp butter or coconut oil

TO SERVE

Greek yoghurt, extra blueberries, honey and cinnamon

1 Put the chopped banana in a bowl and mash it with a fork. Add the egg, milk, oat bran or protein powder and the cinnamon and beat everything together until smooth. Set the mixture aside for 5 minutes to allow the oat bran or protein powder to be absorbed, then fold in the blueberries and seeds.

2 Heat a frying pan over a medium heat for a minute or so. Add the butter or coconut oil and let it melt. As soon as it's melted, drop spoonfuls of the batter into the pan – 3 or 4 will probably be enough as the pancakes expand as they cook. Once the pancakes are golden underneath, flip them over and cook them on the other side, again until golden.

3 Remove the pancakes from the pan, put them on a plate and keep them warm while you make the rest.

4 Serve the pancakes with a dollop of yoghurt, some extra blueberries, a drizzle of honey (a teaspoonful is plenty) and a pinch of cinnamon.

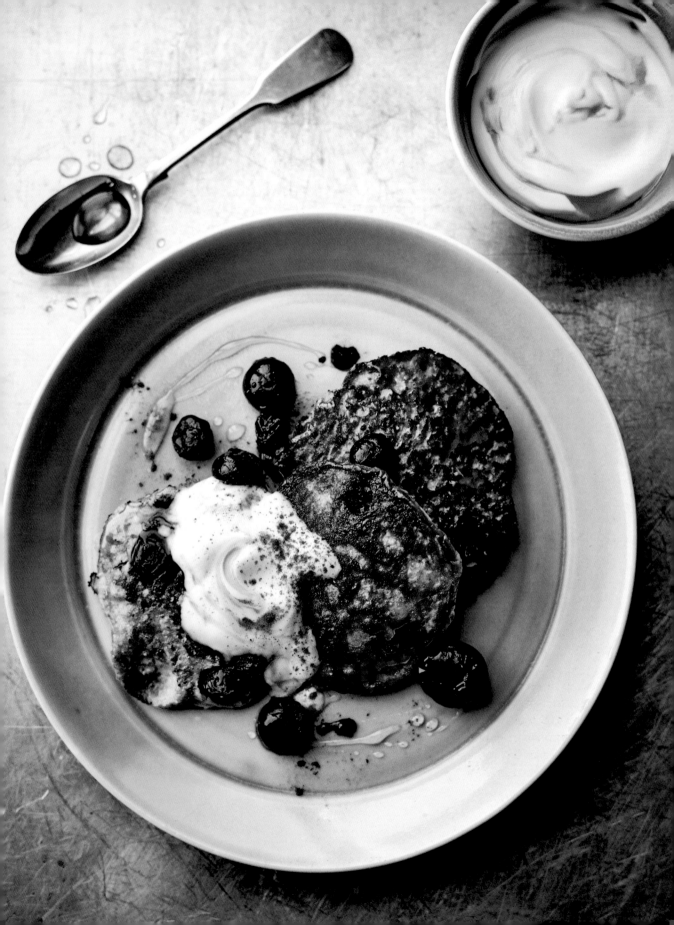

≈ CHEESY RICOTTA AND ≈ HERB PANCAKES

I love the creamy taste of ricotta and these savoury, extra-fluffy pancakes are light and really delicious. The batter doesn't need to rest so you can use it straight away, making this great option if you're short of time.

MAKES 8 PANCAKES

79 CALORIES PER PANCAKE

2 medium eggs, separated

100g ricotta

20g Parmesan cheese, finely grated

1 tbsp wholemeal flour

2 tbsp freshly chopped herbs, such as chives, dill or parsley – or use a mixture

1 tsp olive oil

salt and freshly ground black pepper

TO SERVE

a few tomatoes, sliced or ½ avocado, sliced

small handful of rocket leaves

1 Put the egg yolks, ricotta, Parmesan, flour and herbs into a bowl. Season with salt and black pepper and mix everything together well.

2 Whisk the egg whites in a scrupulously clean, grease-free bowl until the mixture stands in soft peaks.

3 Fold a spoonful of the beaten egg whites into the ricotta mixture to loosen it, then fold in the remaining egg whites.

4 Heat half the oil in a frying pan over a medium heat. Using a dessertspoon, drop 3 or 4 spoonfuls of the batter into the pan. Once the pancakes are golden on one side turn them over and cook for 1–2 minutes on the other side. Remove the pancakes from the pan and keep them warm.

5 Heat the rest of the oil and cook the remaining mixture – you should have 8–10 pancakes. Serve them with a salad of tomatoes or avocado and some rocket.

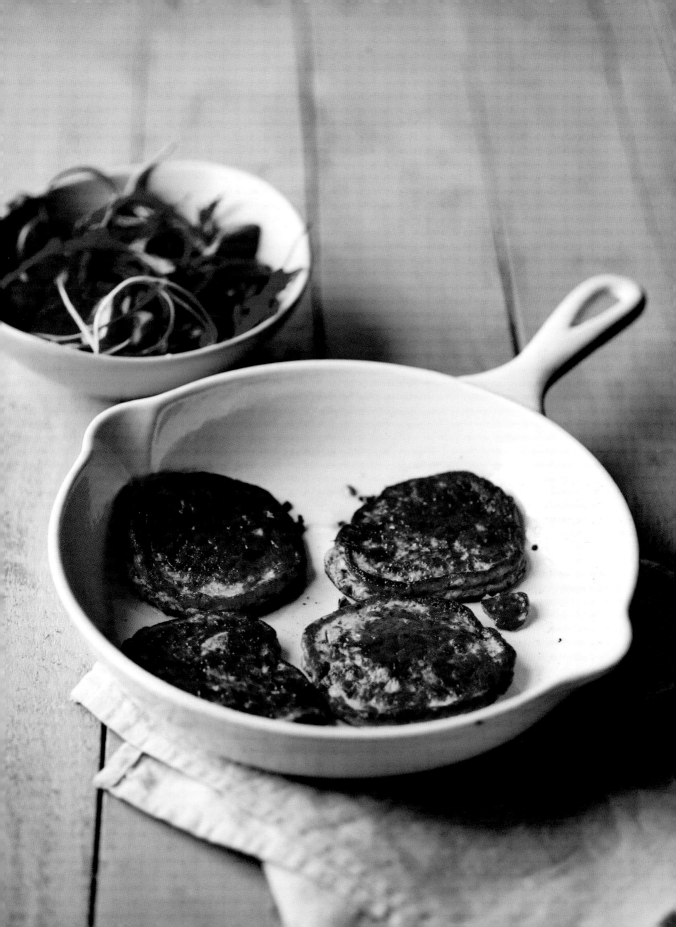

≈ BAKED BREAKFAST MUFFINS ≈
WITH CRISPY 'FRIED' BREAD

These baked eggs are really fun and make a great weekend breakfast or brunch. They are simple to make, look amazing and will kick-start your day. The 'fried' bread cooked alongside the vegetables is lovely and crispy and much healthier than the regular sort.

SERVES 2

527 CALORIES PER SERVING

2 tsp olive oil

4 rashers of streaky bacon, trimmed of any fat

4 medium eggs

2 tomatoes, cut in half

100g chestnut mushrooms

2 sprigs of thyme

4 slices of wholemeal bread

salt and freshly ground black pepper

1 Preheat the oven to 200°C/180°C Fan/ Gas 6.

2 Brush 4 holes of a muffin tin with the olive oil. Place a rasher of bacon into each hole, with one end covering the base and the rest wrapped around the sides.

3 Crack an egg into each bacon-lined hole in the muffin tin. Season the eggs with salt and pepper.

4 Put the tomatoes and mushrooms in a small roasting tin and season them with salt and pepper. Drizzle them with a little oil and scatter over the thyme. Cut out 4 rounds of bread from the slices with a 7cm scone cutter or a glass of a similar size, brush them with the remaining olive oil and put them in the roasting tin too.

5 Put the muffin tin on the highest shelf in the oven and the roasting tin on the shelf below. Cook for 15–20 minutes until the eggs have set and the vegetables are tender. Serve each of the egg muffins on the crisp 'fried' bread with the vegetables alongside.

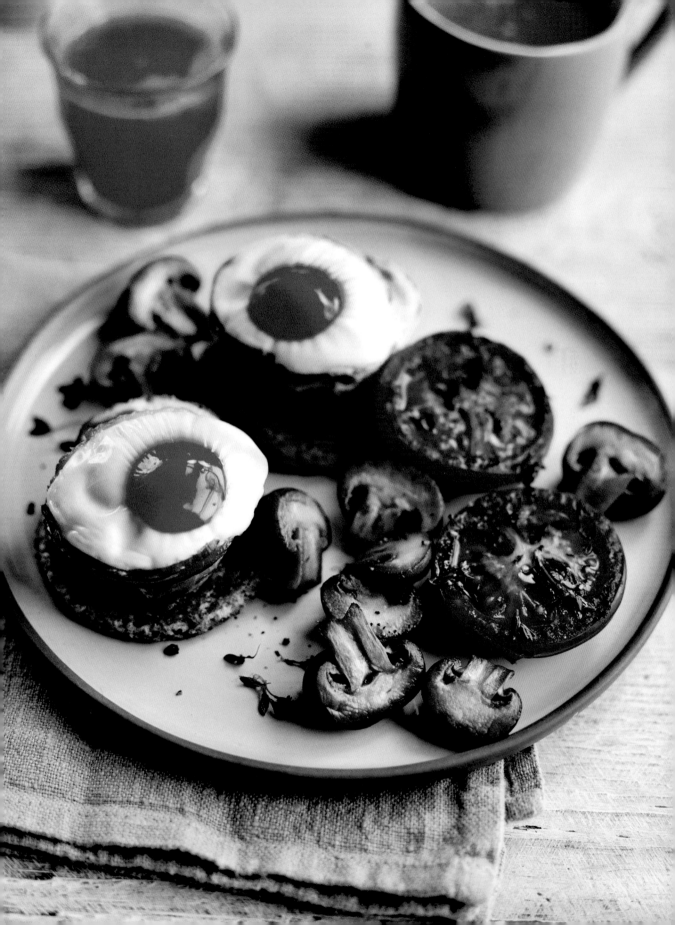

≈ SCRAMBLED EGGS ≈ TOM'S WAY

For me, eggs are the perfect breakfast. They taste great, are easy to cook and are packed full of protein and good fats to keep me going all morning. This is my favourite scrambled eggs recipe and it includes some veg for extra goodness.

SERVES 2

319 CALORIES PER SERVING

6 eggs

15g butter

1 large tomato, finely chopped

150g spinach, washed

a few sprigs of parsley, finely chopped

salt and freshly ground black pepper

1 Beat the eggs in a bowl and season them well. Pour them into a medium non-stick saucepan and place the pan over a gentle heat. Start stirring as soon as the eggs begin to cook around the sides.

2 Meanwhile, melt half the butter in a separate pan over a gentle heat. Add the tomato, season well and cook for a minute or so to soften. Add the spinach, then cover the pan with a lid so that the spinach steams in the heat.

3 Check the eggs and give them a final really good stir to make sure they're well scrambled. Stir in the rest of the butter.

4 Spoon the eggs on to plates and add the spinach and tomatoes. Scatter over the parsley and serve at once.

TOM'S TIP

I like my scrambled eggs with a couple of slices of lean ham on the side too. About 25–50g is enough, depending on how hungry you are, and use just 4 eggs because there is already protein in the ham. For something a bit different, finely slice a couple of spring onions and scatter half over each serving, then sprinkle with chia seeds or linseeds – half a teaspoon on each plate.

≈

≈ BOILED EGGS ≈
WITH SPICED PITTA DIPPERS

Eggs and soldiers were a favourite of mine when I was a child. Nowadays, I like to turn this classic into something more exciting with these spicy dippers. You can adjust the amount of spice to suit your taste buds – just a hint or hot, hot, hot!

SERVES 2

291 CALORIES PER SERVING

10g softened butter

good pinch or 2 each of paprika, turmeric, ground cumin and ground coriander

4 medium eggs, at room temperature

1 pitta bread, sliced into fingers

salt and freshly ground black pepper

1 In a small bowl, mix together the butter and spices – add a pinch of each spice, then taste and add more if you like. Season with salt and pepper.

2 Preheat the grill and bring a medium saucepan of water to the boil. Once the water is boiling, carefully lower the eggs into the pan. Cook them for 4–5 minutes for soft yolks.

3 Meanwhile, grill the pitta fingers on one side, then spread a little of the spicy butter over each of them. Serve the pitta fingers with the boiled eggs and enjoy dipping them into the golden yolks.

≈ SPINACH AND EGGS ≈

Blending a delicious combination of nutritious ingredients, this great one-pan dish is the ultimate pick-me-up breakfast or brunch. It's topped with a tasty dressing made from yoghurt with a hint of mustard, but if you don't fancy mustard first thing, just stir in a squeeze of lemon juice instead.

SERVES 2

300 CALORIES PER SERVING

1 tsp olive oil

10g butter

1 shallot, finely sliced

125g spinach, washed and chopped

125g kale, washed and finely chopped

60g frozen peas, thawed

grating of nutmeg

4 medium eggs

salt and freshly ground black pepper

TO SERVE

2 tbsp plain yoghurt

1 tsp wholegrain mustard or a squeeze of lemon juice

1 Heat the oil and butter in a frying pan over a medium heat. Add the shallot and cook it for 3 minutes until it starts to soften.

2 Stir in the spinach, kale and peas, season well and add a little grated nutmeg. Cook for 2 more minutes until the greens start to wilt down.

3 Make 4 holes in the spinach mixture and crack an egg into each hole. Put a lid on the pan, turn the heat down low and leave the eggs to cook until the whites are set but the yolks are still soft.

4 Whisk the yoghurt and the mustard or lemon juice with a tablespoon of water and season with salt and pepper. Serve the eggs and greens on to plates, then spoon the yoghurt dressing on top. Eat at once!

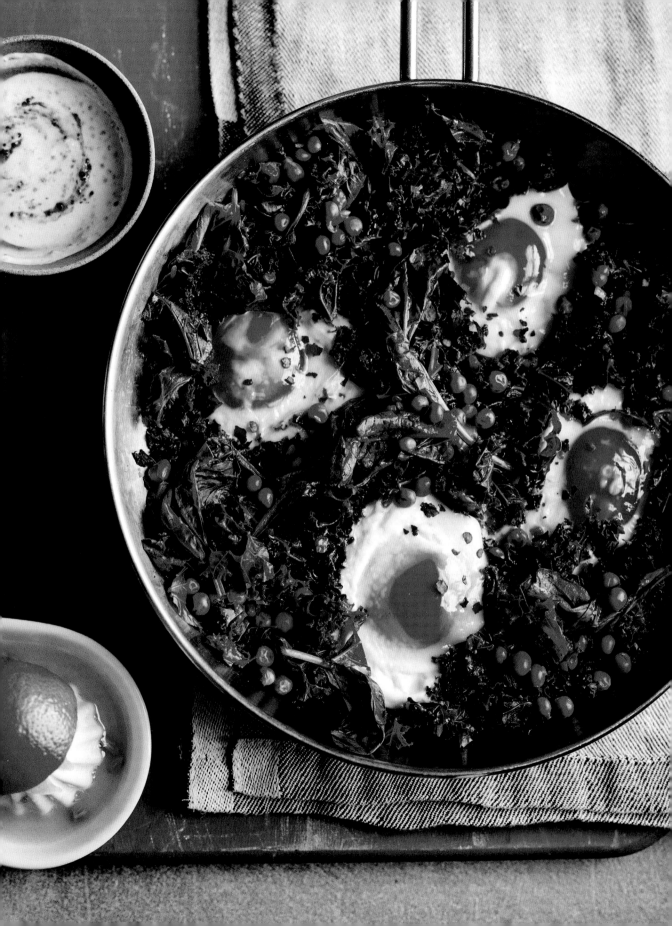

≈ THE ULTIMATE BACON BUTTY ≈

I have to confess that when I'm in the mood for a bacon sarnie, nothing else will do. Here's a healthy twist on the classic butty that really hits the spot.

SERVES 2

290 CALORIES PER SERVING

1 tbsp mixed seeds, such as pumpkin and linseed

2 rashers of back bacon, trimmed of fat

2 plum or medium beef tomatoes, halved

½ large avocado

pinch of chilli flakes

good squeeze of lemon juice

2 slices of sourdough bread

salt and freshly ground black pepper

1 Toast the seeds in a dry frying pan until golden, tossing them frequently.

2 Preheat the grill until hot and grill the bacon and tomatoes until the bacon is cooked, turning it once, and the tomatoes have softened.

3 Mash the avocado flesh in a bowl, then stir in the chilli and lemon juice. Season well and mix again.

4 Toast the bread, then divide the avocado between the slices. Top with tomatoes and bacon, sprinkle over the seeds and serve.

TOM'S TIP

This recipe is for open sandwiches, but if you're really hungry – like me – add another slice of toast on top! This will add about 100 extra calories.

≈

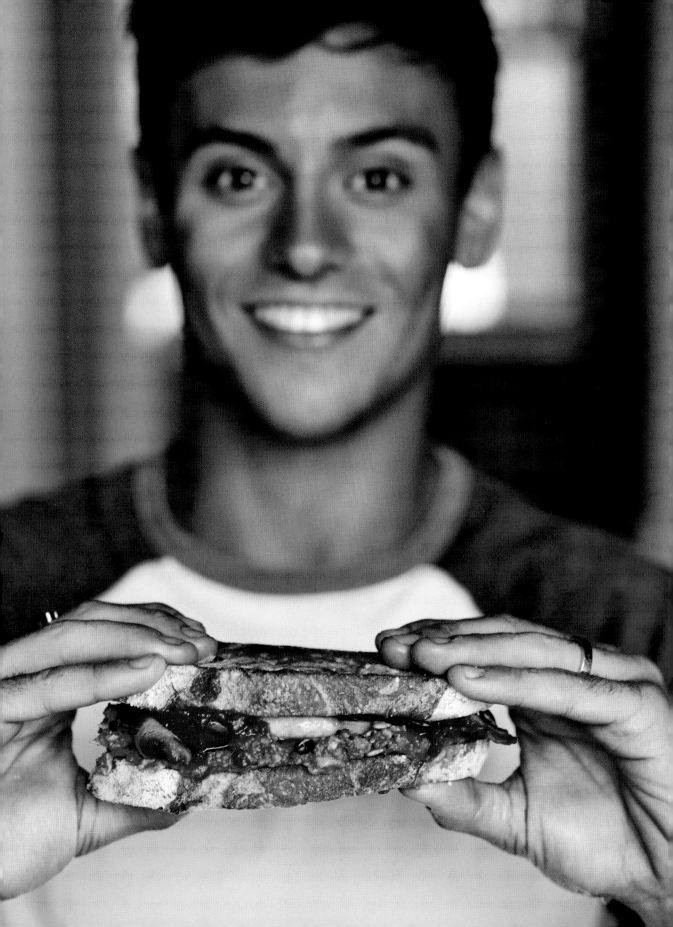

~ QUICK HOME-MADE BEANS ~
WITH HEALTHY 'FRIED' EGGS

I love beans for breakfast and they're packed full of energy. This recipe makes a generous amount of beans for two but could stretch to four with extra side dishes. The eggs are cooked in a non-stick pan with water so they steam rather than fry.

SERVES 2, GENEROUSLY

456 CALORIES PER SERVING

1 tsp olive oil

1 shallot, finely chopped

400g can of chopped tomatoes

200ml hot vegetable or chicken stock

1 sprig of rosemary

1 bay leaf

1 tbsp sun-dried tomato paste

400g can of cannellini beans, drained

2 eggs

2 slices of sourdough bread

butter

salt and freshly ground black pepper

1 Heat the oil in a saucepan and cook the shallot over a medium heat for 3–4 minutes until softened.

2 Add the chopped tomatoes, stock, herbs and tomato paste to the pan and bring to the boil. Season with salt and pepper, then stir everything together and simmer for 12–15 minutes until the sauce has reduced and thickened.

3 Stir in the cannellini beans and continue to simmer for a couple of minutes to warm them through.

4 Heat 2 tablespoons of water in a non-stick frying pan. As soon as the water is boiling and has reduced by about half, add the eggs. Turn the heat down low and cover the pan with a lid. Cook the eggs for about 3 minutes until the whites have set and the yolks are still soft.

5 Toast the slices of sourdough bread and spread them with a little butter. Put the toast on plates, divide the beans between them and carefully place an egg on top of each serving.

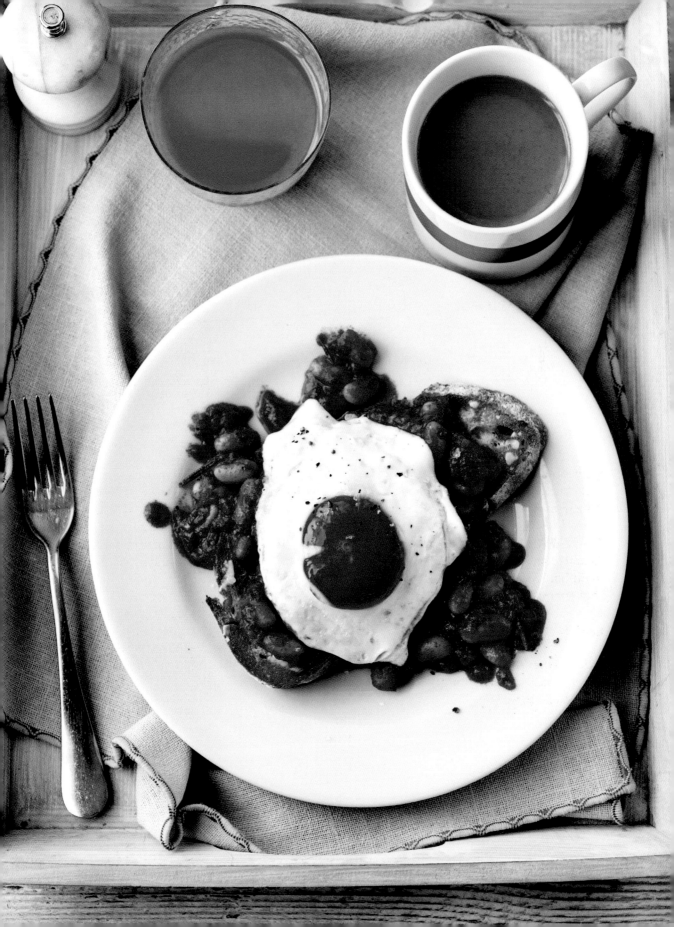

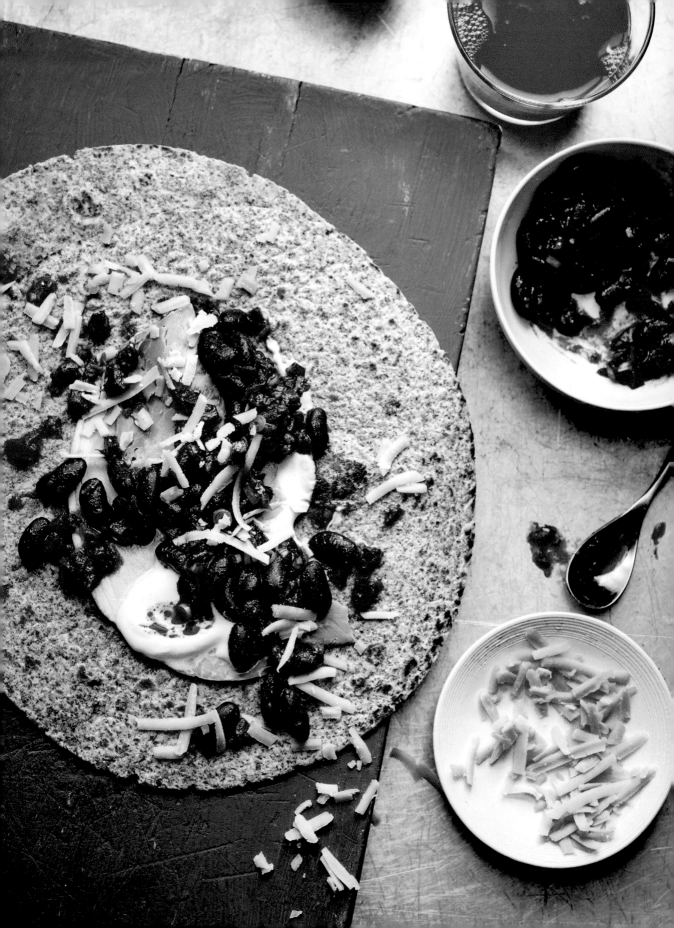

TOASTED
≈ BREAKFAST BURRITOS ≈

These breakfast burrito bundles are a real feast and give you an energy-filled start to the day. They're good with ham, or see my tips for egg or bacon burritos below. The salsa is really good and goes brilliantly with my fabulous fajitas too (see page 128).

SERVES 2

384 CALORIES PER SERVING

½ can of kidney beans, drained

2 wholemeal tortilla wraps

2 slices of ham (about 60g)

2 tbsp Greek yoghurt

20g mature Cheddar cheese, grated

salt and freshly ground black pepper

SALSA

2 tomatoes (about 100g), deseeded and chopped

1 spring onion, chopped

¼ pepper, deseeded and chopped

1 tsp tomato purée

½ tsp olive oil

1 For the salsa, put the tomatoes, spring onion, pepper, tomato purée and oil into a small blender and whizz to chop the veg finely and make a nice chunky mixture.

2 Tip half the salsa into a bowl and season well, then stir in the kidney beans. You can store the rest of the salsa in a sealable container in the fridge for up to 4 days.

3 Lay the tortillas on a board and put a slice of ham on each. Add a spoonful of yoghurt, then top with the bean mixture and sprinkle over the cheese. Season again.

4 Roll the burritos up, then wrap each one in foil. Heat a frying pan, place the foil parcels in it and toast the burritos for a couple of minutes all over.

VARIATIONS

SCRAMBLED EGG BURRITO

404 CALORIES PER SERVING

Scramble an egg in a separate pan and spoon it on to the ham instead of the yoghurt. Follow the rest of the recipe as before.

BACON BURRITO

378 CALORIES PER SERVING

Cook 2 rashers of back bacon, trimmed of any fat, in a pan until golden. Lay the bacon rashers on the tortilla, instead of the ham and Greek yoghurt, then follow the rest of the recipe as before.

~ KEDGEREE WITH SALMON ~

I'm happy to eat this warm and comforting breakfast dish at any time of day, but it is a perfect brunch. It's usually made with smoked haddock, but my version uses salmon instead and tastes amazing. Including some grated courgette means you don't need so much rice and keeps this low carb.

SERVES 2

495 CALORIES PER SERVING

200g salmon fillet

1 tbsp olive oil

2 large spring onions, sliced into small rings

¾ tsp curry powder

¼ tsp turmeric

good pinch of chilli flakes

75g brown basmati rice

275ml hot vegetable or chicken stock

1 small courgette, finely grated

60g frozen peas, thawed

2 eggs

2 tbsp parsley, plus extra to garnish

salt and freshly ground black pepper

1 Preheat the grill. Season the salmon fillet with salt and pepper and grill it for about 10 minutes until cooked. Set the fish aside until it's cool enough to handle, then flake it into large chunks.

2 Heat the oil in a saucepan and stir-fry the spring onions for 2–3 minutes until softened. Stir in the spices and season well, then continue to stir-fry for a minute or so to cook the spices.

3 Stir in the rice and cook for 1 minute to coat it in the spices. Pour the hot stock over the top and put a lid on the pan. Bring the stock to the boil, then turn the heat down low and cook for 20–25 minutes.

4 Take the lid off the pan and quickly spoon the grated courgette and peas on top of the rice. Cover the pan again and continue to cook for 3–5 minutes longer until all the water has been absorbed and the courgette and peas are tender.

5 Meanwhile, bring a small pan of water to the boil and cook the eggs for 6 minutes. Drain well and cover the eggs with cold water, then carefully peel off the shells.

6 Fluff up the rice and stir in the parsley and salmon flakes, then divide the kedgeree between 2 bowls. Halve the eggs, arrange them on top and scatter over a little more parsley if you like before serving.

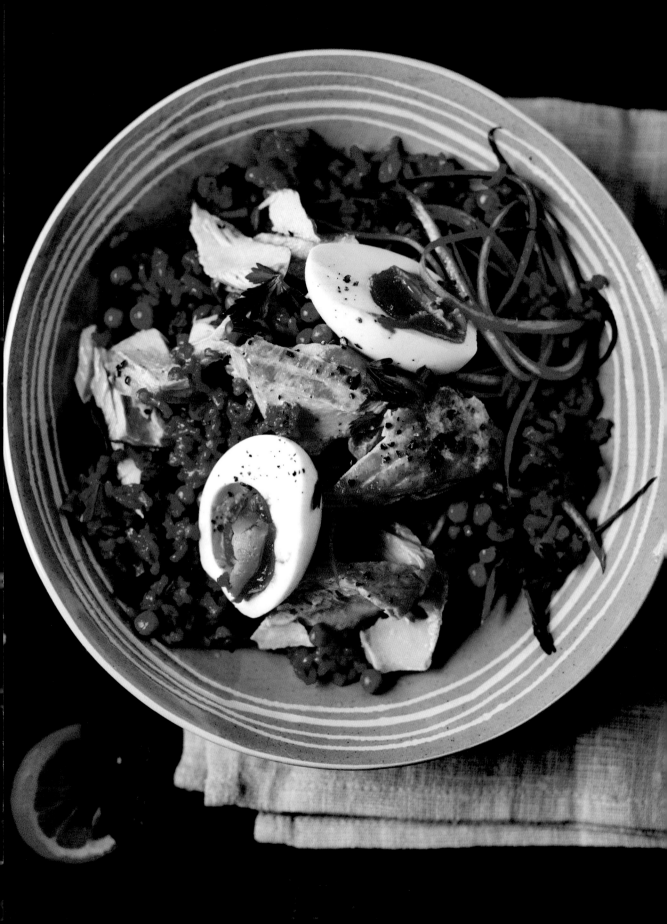

≈ TOMS'S BIG FRY-UP ≈

I love a good fry-up and this hearty full English, with a few changes to cut
the fat, will help you build strength, keep hunger at bay and make the most
of a weekend morning. Make sure you remove all visible fat from the
bacon and use high-meat-content sausages.

SERVES 2

516 CALORIES PER SERVING

2 sausages

2 rashers of bacon

drizzle of olive oil

2 eggs

1 plum tomato, halved

½ quantity home-made beans
(see p. 26) or ½ can baked beans

SWEET POTATO ROSTI

1 tsp olive oil

200g sweet potato, grated

2 spring onions, chopped

1 large egg, beaten

2 tbsp freshly chopped parsley

couple of splashes of
Worcestershire sauce (optional)

salt and freshly ground
black pepper

1 Heat a large frying pan (or use a Master Pan) until hot and add the sausages. Cook them for about 15 minutes, turning them regularly until golden brown. Add the rashers of bacon to the pan after about 10 minutes and cook them until they're golden and crisp.

2 Add a drizzle of oil to the pan and fry the eggs, trying to keep the white to one side only and leaving space for the tomato. Cook until the whites are set and the yolks are done to your liking. You may find it useful to put a lid on the pan at this stage to help the eggs cook. Add the tomato, cut-side down, tucking it in around the sausages and bacon. Heat the baked beans in a separate pan.

3 While the sausages and bacon are cooking, make the rosti. Heat the oil in a separate medium frying pan. Mix together the grated sweet potato, spring onions, egg, parsley and Worcestershire sauce, if using, and season well. Spoon the mixture into the heated frying pan and squash it down with the back of a spoon until it covers the base. Cook for about 4 minutes until the mixture is golden underneath.

4 Slide the rosti on to a plate, then flip it over and back into the pan to cook the other side. If you find this difficult, just flip pieces of rosti over in the pan and squash them back together again. Cook for a further 4 minutes, again until golden underneath. Alternatively, divide the mixture roughly into 4 and cook as smaller rostis, following the method above.

5 Slice the rosti in half and put half on each plate. Serve the sausages, bacon, tomatoes, eggs and beans too and tuck in.

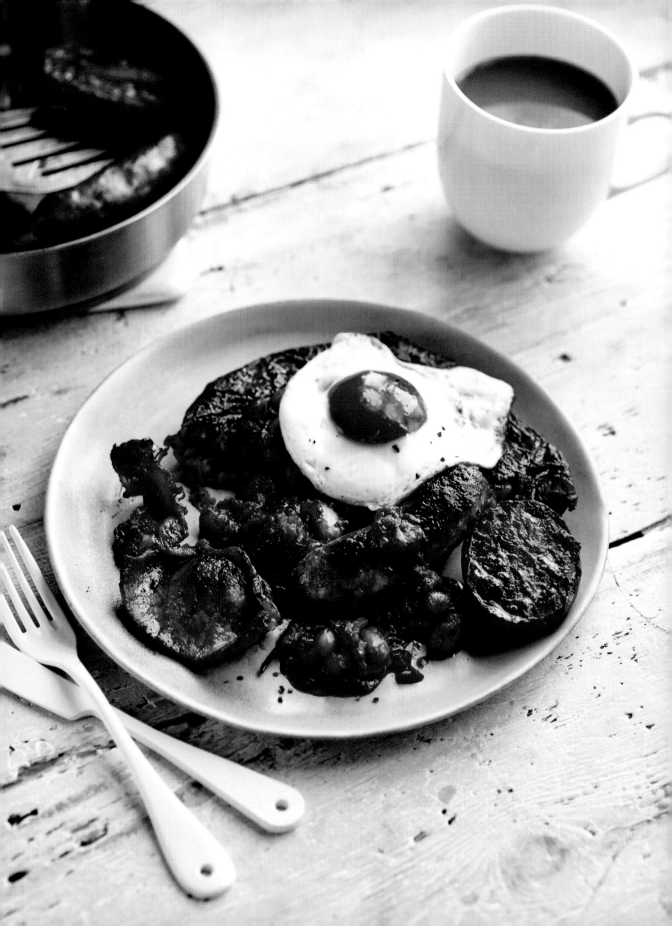

≈ SIMPLE PORRIDGE ≈

Porridge is my go-to fitness food and on cold mornings there's nothing I like better than this comforting breakfast classic. Loaded with fibre and packed with vitamins and minerals, porridge is great plain or with one of my topping ideas.

SERVES 2

400 CALORIES PER SERVING

80g porridge oats

500ml whole milk

TOPPING

1 tbsp flaked almonds

1 small apple, cored and grated

squeeze of orange juice

1 Put the flaked almonds in a frying pan and toast them gently over a medium heat for 2–3 minutes, tossing them every now and then, until they are lightly browned. Mix the toasted almonds with the rest of the topping ingredients and set aside.

2 Put the oats and milk in a saucepan and place the pan over a medium heat. Slowly bring the milk to the boil, then keep stirring until the oats are cooked and the mixture is thick and creamy.

3 Serve the porridge with the apple and almond mixture – or with one of the toppings below.

VARIATIONS

FIG AND PECAN TOPPING

460 CALORIES PER SERVING

Chop 2 dried figs and 10 pecan nuts. Scatter them over the porridge, then sprinkle a little cinnamon on top.

MANGO AND COCONUT TOPPING

385 CALORIES PER SERVING

Chop half a fresh mango into cubes and add them to the porridge, then scatter over 2 teaspoons of toasted unsweetened desiccated coconut.

TOM'S TIP
Try a spoonful of my peanut and cashew butter (p.172) on your porridge for an extra treat.

~ TOAST-IN-THE-PAN GRANOLA ~

Ready-made granola is a handy store-cupboard breakfast, but I've realised that the packaged versions often contain lots of sugar. This is a quick, easy and tempting alternative – and you don't even need to turn on the oven!

MAKES ABOUT 12 SERVINGS

266 CALORIES PER SERVING (WITHOUT MILK OR YOGHURT)

3 tbsp coconut oil

1½ tsp ground mixed spice

3 tbsp thick honey

220g oats

50g brazil nuts, roughly chopped

50g whole almonds, roughly chopped

35g cashew nuts

20g pumpkin seeds

15g sunflower seeds

50g apricots, chopped

50g sultanas

TO SERVE

milk, plain yoghurt, fruit

1 Heat the oil in a large wok over a medium heat and add the spice and honey. Cook for 1 minute, stirring all the ingredients together until they're hot and bubbling.

2 Add the remaining ingredients and cook for 8–10 minutes until everything is toasted and bits are starting to stick together. Toss the mixture every now and then to check that the underneath isn't burning.

3 Take the pan off the heat and transfer the mixture to a container. Leave it to cool. You'll find that once the mixture has cooled it will stick together in little clumps like traditional granola. When the granola is completely cool put a lid on the container. Eat within a couple of weeks.

4 To serve, put 50g of granola in a bowl, add milk and top with some plain yoghurt and fruit.

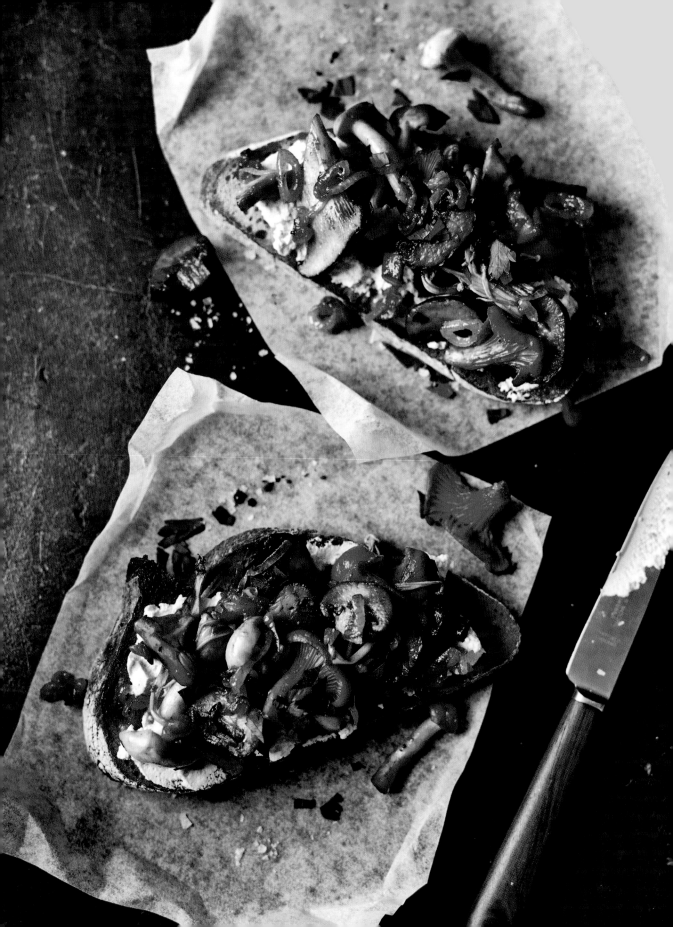

≈ MUSHROOMS ≈
ON TOAST

Something on toast is always a treat and this tasty breakfast takes just moments to make. It's extra good with chestnut or wild mushrooms, but the button kind work fine too. The ricotta is delicious, but you could also use cream cheese or cottage cheese.

SERVES 2

182 CALORIES PER SERVING

10g butter

1 shallot, finely sliced

300g mixed mushrooms (chestnut and wild), sliced if large

1 tbsp freshly chopped parsley

2 slices of sourdough or grainy bread

2 tbsp ricotta

salt and freshly ground black pepper

1 Melt the butter in a small frying pan and cook the shallot over a medium heat for 3–4 minutes until it's starting to soften.

2 Stir in the mushrooms and add a tablespoon of water to the pan. Season the mushrooms well, then stir-fry them for 1 minute. Cover the pan with a lid and cook the mushrooms for 3–4 minutes more until they are done all the way through. Stir in the chopped parsley.

3 Toast the bread and spread a tablespoon of ricotta over each slice. Put the toast on plates, spoon the mushrooms on top and season again, then eat at once.

TOM'S TIP
I love chilli and I sometimes sprinkle a few chilli flakes over the mushrooms to give them a bit of a kick.

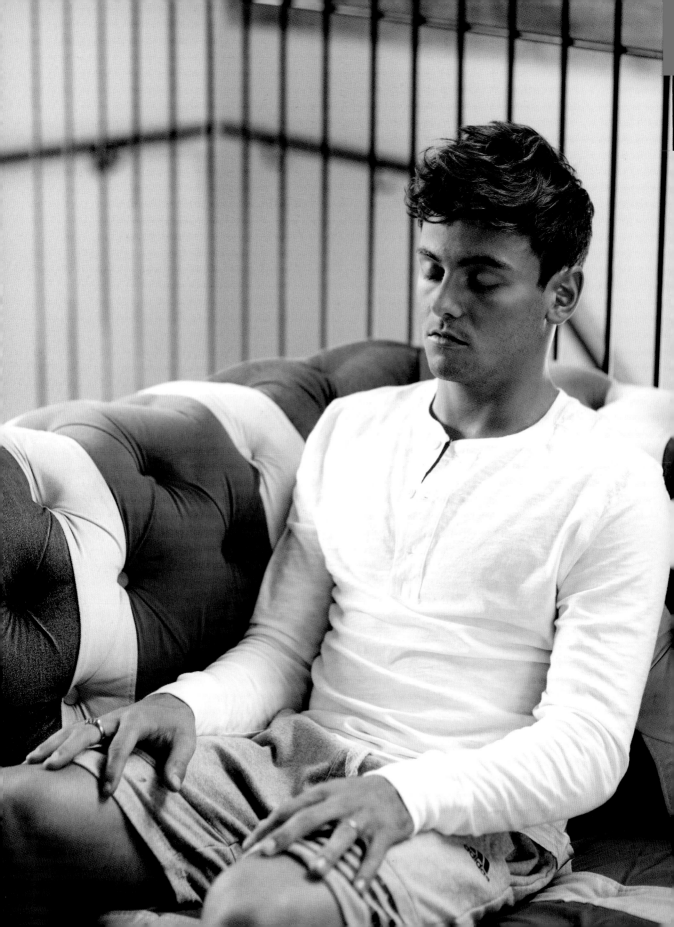

MORNING LIFE HACKS
≈ MEDITATION ≈

You might think meditation is not for you. I wasn't too sure at first, but I started meditating in 2013 and now I'm hooked. Most mornings I like to get up early enough to eat a proper breakfast and to meditate. Then I head off for training feeling calm, focused and rested. Here's a ten-minute meditation exercise you could do at home before you start your day. It's so worth it.

1 Find a quiet spot and sit comfortably on a chair with a straight back.

2 Shut the door, set an alarm if you like and try to make sure you'll be left undisturbed for ten minutes.

3 Close your eyes. Take three deep breaths, inhaling through your nose and breathing out through your mouth.

4 Focus on the physical sensations in your body. Think about how your feet feel against the floor and your back against the chair. Can you feel your abdomen rise and fall with each breath you take?

5 From your head downwards, scan through your body, working down to your feet. Notice the feelings you have: which parts feel relaxed, tight or numb? Note the sensations but don't try to change them.

6 Once you've scanned right down to the tips of your toes, come back to focusing your mind. Notice your breath and how it feels. Count ten breaths. If thoughts come into your mind, just bring your attention back to your breath.

7 Now turn your thoughts to your body. Count to three and then gently open your eyes when you feel ready. All done!

MORNING LIFE HACKS
≈ SETTING GOALS ≈

Do you ever think about where you want to be in one month, one year or five years' time? I know – there's more than enough to think about every day without that, but setting goals can help you grow in ways you might not have imagined. So whether you want to improve your fitness, get a promotion or simply have more adventures in life, here are my goal-setting tips.

HAVE GOALS THAT MOTIVATE YOU

Set goals that have a high priority in your life, so you are committed to maximising your chance of success. If your goals are important to you, there's value in achieving them.

SET ACHIEVABLE GOALS

Break down your ultimate goal into steps that are easy to achieve. For example, if you want to lose a stone in weight, start by aiming to lose one or two pounds a week through healthy eating and exercise. Shedding a stone might seem impossible but a pound or two you can manage. An achievable goal makes it easier to stay on track, reach your targets and experience the thrill of success. This all helps to spur you on to reach your ultimate goal.

CHECK YOUR PROGRESS

It's easy to become so focused on the outcome that you forget all the small steps needed to get there. Write these steps down and cross them off as you complete them, so you can see you're making progress

VISUALISE SUCCESS

Before you can really believe you can achieve something, you need a clear idea of what it might look like. When you visualise your goal, you can begin to 'see' the possibility of achieving it. Take that moment and feeling and run with it! It will help to make you more motivated and prepared to make sacrifices to achieve your target.

MAKE THE TIME

Goal setting is more than just saying you *want* to do something. Most of us have a routine in our lives and it's important to build in the time for whatever it is you want to achieve so it actually does happen.

WHEN YOU VISUALISE YOUR GOAL, YOU BEGIN TO 'SEE' THE POSSIBILITY OF ACHIEVING IT

MORNING LIFE HACKS
≈ MANAGING YOUR TIME ≈

We all lead such busy lives and I often used to find myself saying 'I'm too busy' as an excuse for not doing something. Do you feel you don't have time for exercise, to meet up with old friends or to cook a healthy meal? Here are some tips that I've picked up about time management that you might find helpful too.

PRIORITISE

Think about what you want to achieve on a daily basis and decide on your priorities. Choose your top five tasks and work at them in order of importance. They don't all have to be chores. On a weekend, your priorities might be doing some exercise, calling your mum or doing some grocery shopping so you can cook meals for the week ahead.

GET A GOOD NIGHT'S SLEEP

I like to get nine hours sleep a night when I'm training. I appreciate many people might need less, but cutting out sleep to have more fun or to get more work done is not a great idea because being tired in the day will mean that you can't make the most of your time. Whatever your sleep needs, it's really worth getting to bed early enough to get a good night's sleep.

STOP MULTI-TASKING

Do you find yourself browsing Instagram while you're on the phone? Do you sneak a peek at Facebook during an important meeting? Multi-tasking doesn't work because it lessens productivity. Try to focus on one task at a time and be present in the moment.

LEARN TO SAY 'NO'

Like many people, I find it very hard to say no. We all want to be liked and we don't want to hurt other people's feelings, but saying yes to everything will leave you feeling stressed and without time for the stuff that really matters. If you don't want to do something or simply don't have time for it, say no with conviction. Thank the person for thinking of you, but don't offer maybes or find yourself caught up in excuses and feeling guilty

DON'T PUT THINGS OFF

Is there something important you've been meaning to do for ages but you're putting off? Constantly putting things off makes us feel guilty for what we haven't started. I find it helps me to start the task I've been meaning to do and break it down into manageable steps. Then I tell myself I'm going to spend ten minutes on it, rather than complete the whole thing. I take it step by step and get there in the end.

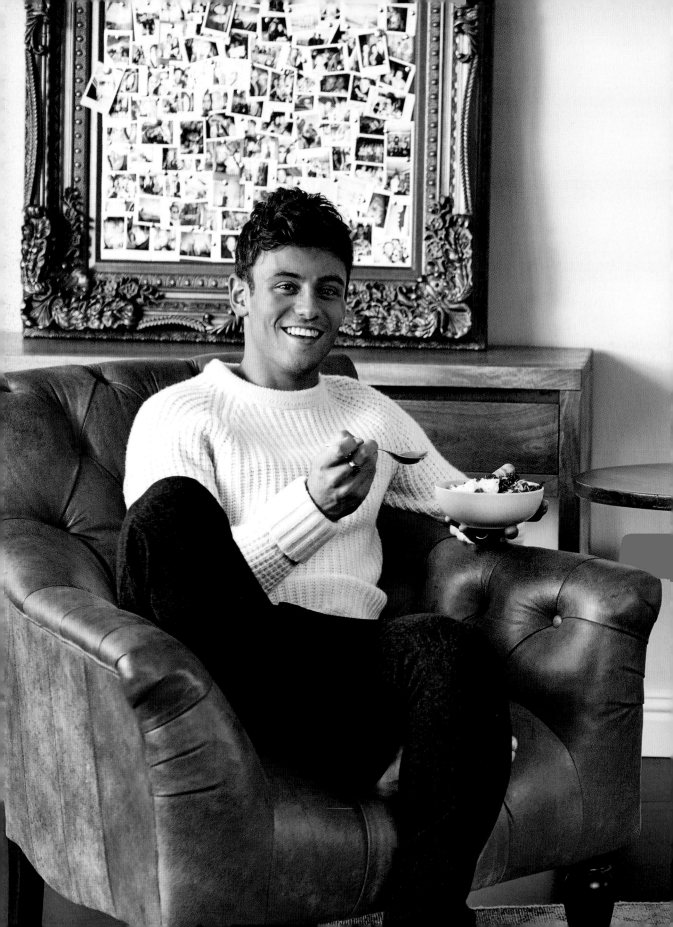

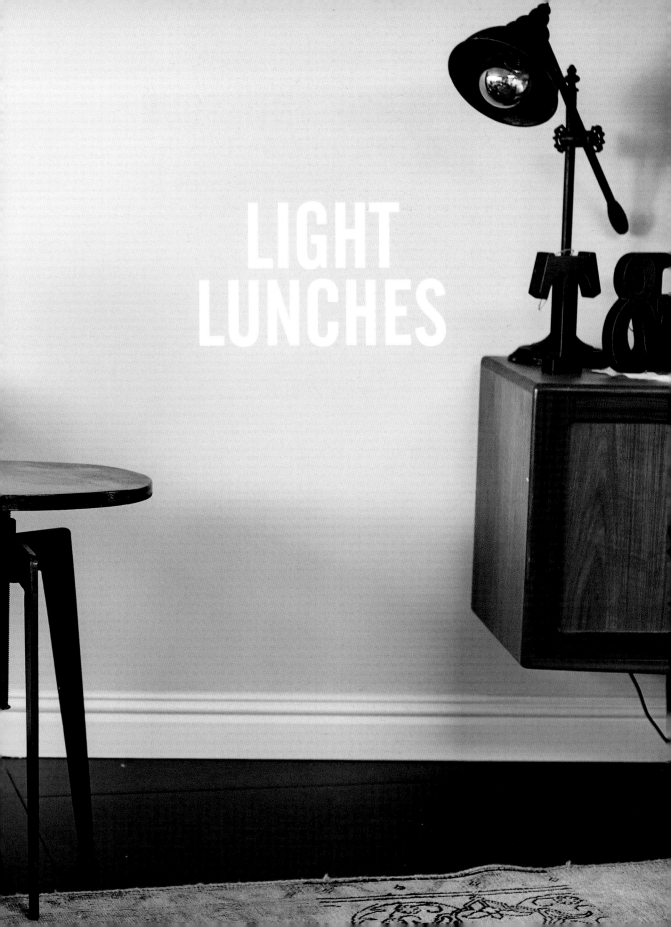

LIGHT
LUNCHES

~ SIMPLE RED LENTIL SOUP ~
WITH CHEESY TORTILLA WEDGES

This low-cost, low-fat soup is really creamy and filling and the tortillas are awesome.
I like to make enough soup for four portions and freeze some for another time.

MAKES 4 SERVINGS

300 CALORIES PER SERVING

1 tbsp olive oil

1 onion, chopped

1 garlic clove, chopped

2 tsp ground coriander

1 tsp ground cumin

½ tsp turmeric

150g red lentils

1 small sweet potato (about 185g), chopped

800ml hot vegetable stock

salt and freshly ground black pepper

CHEESY TORTILLA WEDGES

35g strong Cheddar cheese, grated

1 wholemeal tortilla

½–1 tsp cumin seeds

1 Heat the oil and a tablespoon of water in a saucepan and stir in the onion. Cover the pan with a lid and gently fry the onion for 10–15 minutes over a low heat until it has started to turn golden.

2 Stir in the garlic and spices and cook for 1 minute. Add the red lentils and sweet potato and cook for 2 more minutes. Pour the stock into the pan, cover it with a lid and cook over a low heat for about 15 minutes until the lentils and sweet potato are soft.

3 Preheat the grill. Scatter the cheese over the top of the tortilla and sprinkle with the cumin seeds. Season well, then grill until the cheese is golden and bubbling. There's no need to toast the other side of the tortilla as you want the slices to be nice and soft for dipping in the soup.

4 Whizz the soup with a hand-held blender until smooth, then reheat it gently.

5 Slice the tortilla into thin wedges – a pizza cutter is great for this – and serve them with the soup.

≈
TOM'S TIP
To freeze half this soup, pour it into a sealable container and leave it to cool. Put a lid on the container and freeze the soup for up to a month. When you want to defrost it, leave it in the kitchen overnight, then put it in the fridge until you're ready to heat it up.
≈

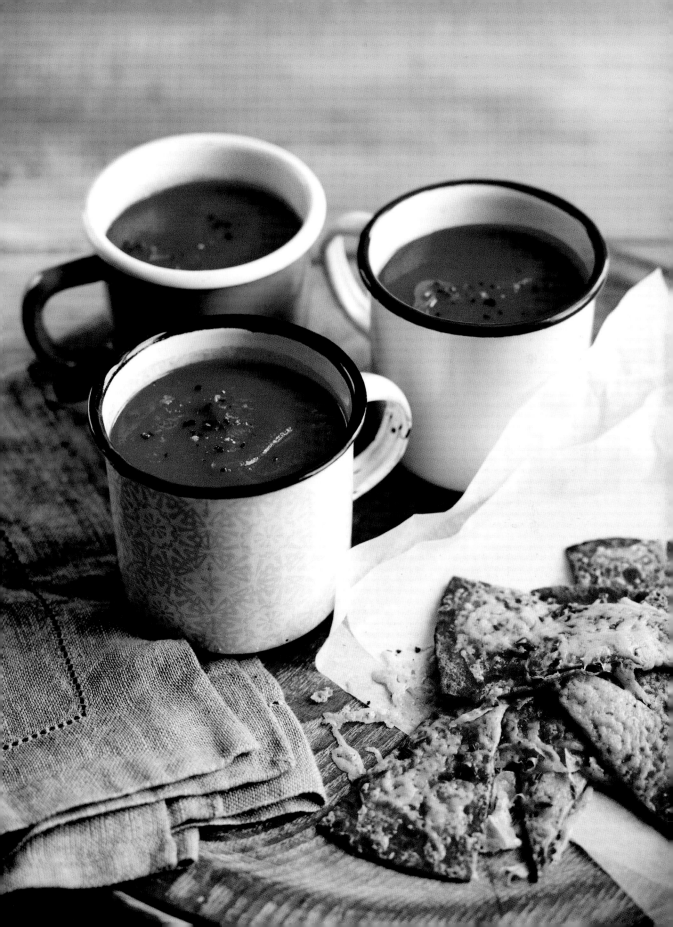

~ ROASTED SQUASH SOUP ~

This hearty soup is simple to make (you don't even need to peel the squash) and makes great comfort food on a cold day. And what's more, you can use any veg you have that might be a bit past its best and the soup will still taste great!

MAKES 4 SERVINGS

114 CALORIES PER SERVING

1 tbsp olive oil

400g butternut squash, unpeeled and cut into chunks

1 red onion, chopped

2 garlic cloves, unpeeled

1 celery stick, roughly chopped

1 carrot, roughly chopped

2 sprigs of thyme

1 tsp smoked paprika

4 slices of pancetta

600ml hot vegetable stock

salt and freshly ground black pepper

1 Preheat the oven to 200°C/180°C Fan/ Gas 6. Put the oil, squash, onion, garlic, celery and carrot in a bowl with the thyme and paprika. Season well and toss everything together. Pour a couple of millimetres of water into a small roasting tin that's large enough to hold the vegetables snugly and in an even layer. Spoon the veg into the tin and roast them for 30 minutes or until tender.

2 Ten minutes before the end of the cooking time, lay the pancetta slices on a piece of baking paper and put them on a baking tray. Pop this into the oven on a shelf below the vegetables and the pancetta should crisp up nicely.

3 When the vegetables are tender, turn off the oven (leave the pancetta in there to keep warm). Tip the vegetables into a food processor. Squeeze the softened garlic out of its skin into the processor, then pull the leaves from the thyme sprigs and add those to the processor too.

4 Add half the stock and whizz until smooth. Tip everything into a pan and add the remaining stock, then bring the soup to a simmer to heat through.

5 Ladle the soup into bowls and top each with some crispy pancetta. Season to taste and serve.

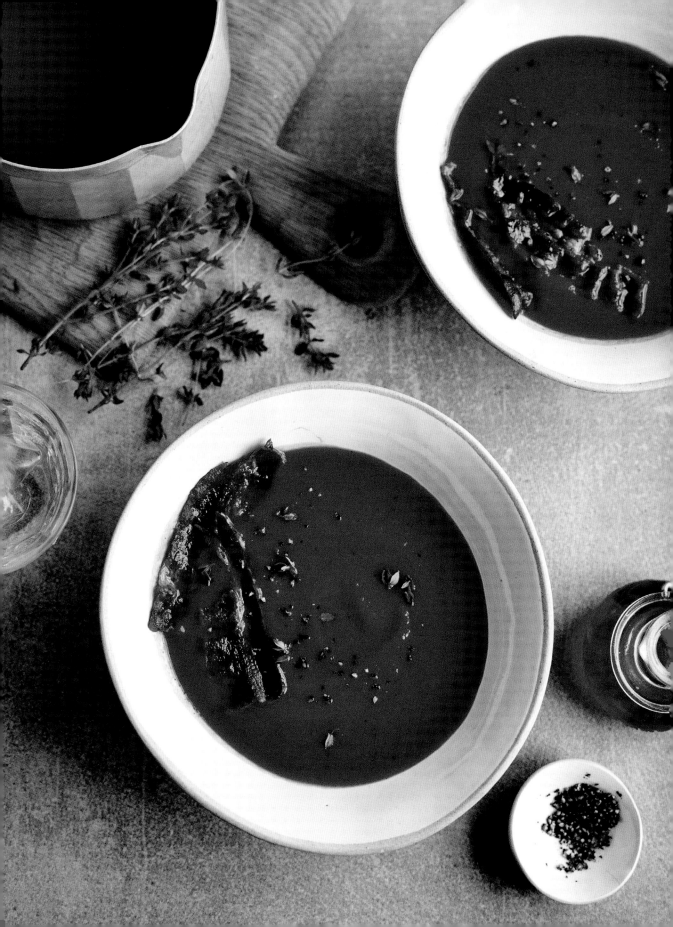

≈ EGG-DROP SOUP ≈

Cracking eggs into hot soup might seem a bit scary, but this tastes brilliant so please do give it a try. Adding the cheese at the end really brings all the flavours together.

SERVES 2

312 CALORIES PER SERVING

1 tbsp olive oil

10g butter

1 leek (about 100g), trimmed, halved, cleaned and sliced

100g savoy cabbage, shredded

300g head of broccoli, chopped

600ml hot vegetable stock

2 large eggs

1 tbsp freshly chopped parsley

15g Parmesan or mature Cheddar cheese

salt and freshly ground black pepper

1 Heat the oil and butter in a saucepan over a low heat. Once the butter has melted, add the leek and savoy cabbage and stir. Season well, then cover the pan with a lid. Cook the vegetables very gently over a low heat for 5 minutes, then add the broccoli and cover the pan again. Cook for another 5–10 minutes until all the vegetables have started to turn golden and caramelise. Stir them every now and then.

2 Stir in the hot stock and season again, then cover the pan and bring the stock to the boil. Turn the heat down low and continue to simmer for 6–8 minutes until the vegetables are tender.

3 Make a dip on one side of the soup with the back of a spoon and drop an egg into it. Do the same on the other side. Cover the pan again and cook for 3 minutes. This method poaches the eggs so that the yolks are set but still a bit soft in the middle.

4 Divide the soup into 2 bowls, making sure there is an egg in each. Scatter over the parsley, then grate half the cheese over each bowlful. Season with pepper, then serve.

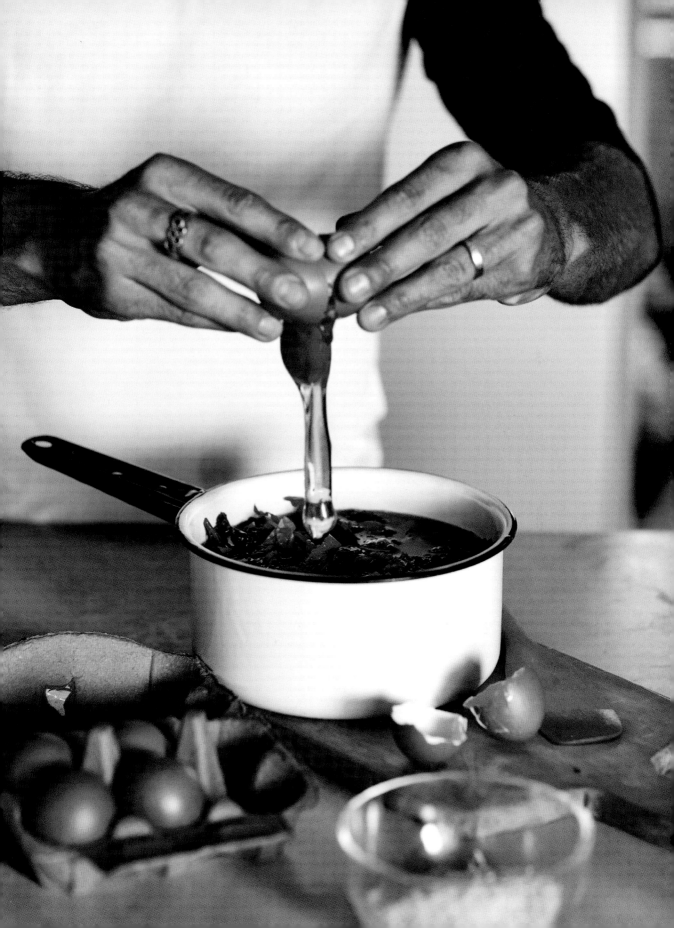

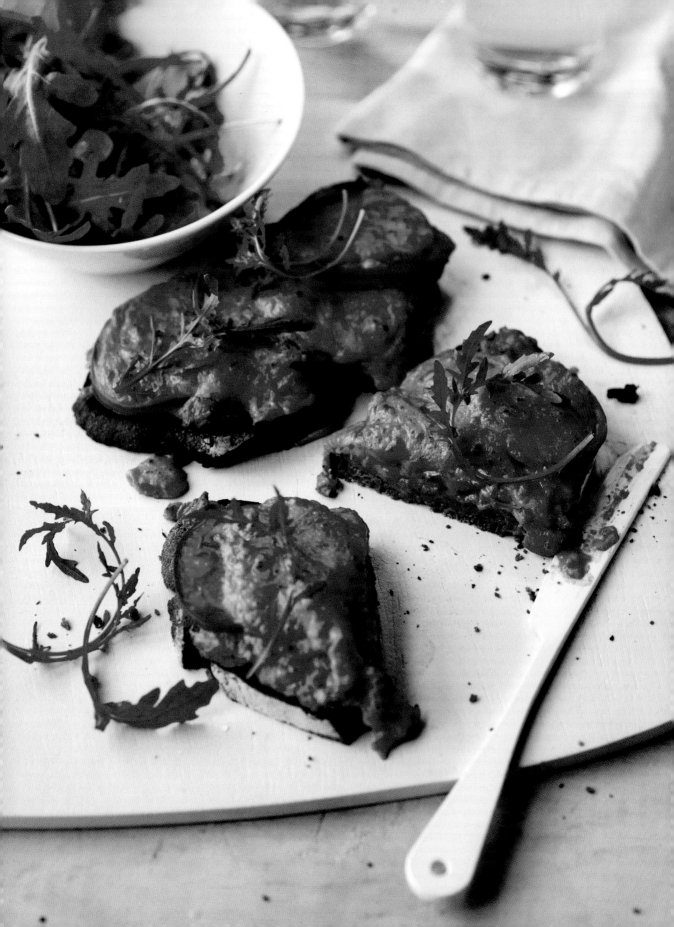

≈ RAREBIT ON RYE ≈

This twist on a classic Welsh rarebit turns cheese on toast into something special. It's simple, satisfying and lower in calories than the traditional recipe. The base is a slice of nutty rye bread, which is first covered with mashed avocado and slices of tomato, before the rarebit mix is spooned on top.

SERVES 2

325 CALORIES PER SERVING

½ avocado

2 slices of rye bread

1 tomato, finely sliced

1 medium egg

1–2 tsp Dijon mustard

50g mature Cheddar cheese, grated

rocket leaves, to serve

salt and freshly ground black pepper

1 Mash the avocado and spread it over the slices of rye bread. Lay the slices of tomato on top. Preheat the grill.

2 Beat the egg, mustard and cheese together in a bowl and season well, then spread this mixture over the tomato.

3 Pop the rarebits under the grill and cook them until they're golden and bubbling.

4 Serve with some rocket leaves scattered over the top.

≈ TOM'S CHICKEN CAESAR SALAD ≈

This is my quick and easy version of the famous Caesar salad and it makes a deliciously light but really satisfying meal. The egg yolk gives the dressing a great creamy texture and there are loads of other awesome flavours.

SERVES 2

380 CALORIES PER SERVING

1 slice of sourdough rye bread (about 30g), chopped into chunks

1 medium egg yolk

1 tsp Dijon mustard (optional)

1 tbsp olive or sunflower oil

15g Parmesan cheese, finely grated

2 anchovy fillets, drained of oil

1 cos lettuce, leaves separated

¼ cucumber, peeled, halved, deseeded and finely sliced

½ avocado, sliced

2 tbsp cress

200g leftover roast chicken, sliced

salt and freshly ground black pepper

1 Preheat the grill. To make crunchy croutons, put the chunks of sourdough on a baking tray and toast them under the grill, turning them every now and then until they're golden all over.

2 Put the egg yolk, mustard, oil, Parmesan and anchovy fillets into a food processor with a tablespoon of cold water. Whizz briefly to make a smooth dressing.

3 Put the lettuce into a large bowl and scatter over the cucumber, avocado and cress. Drizzle over the dressing and toss everything together.

4 Serve the salad in bowls and top with the croutons and slices of chicken.

TOM'S TIP
You can also serve this as a wrap. Leave out the croutons and complete the rest of the recipe as above. Divide the salad between 2 wholemeal wraps, then top with the chicken and enjoy.
≈

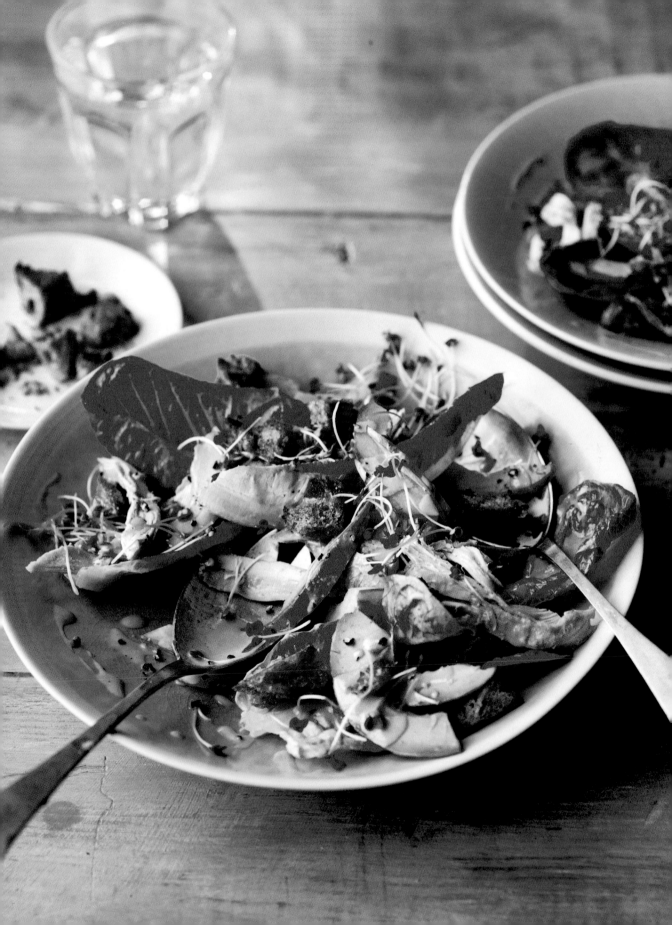

≈ CHICKEN AND MANGO SALAD ≈
WITH NOODLES

Light and fruity, this salad is the perfect dish for warm weather. It's filling too, and it makes an ideal packed lunch. If you want a kick of heat, add a few slices of chilli.

SERVES 2

426 CALORIES PER SERVING

100g buckwheat noodles

60g mangetout, finely sliced

60g green beans or runner beans, finely sliced

60g radishes, finely sliced

½ mango, finely sliced

150g leftover roast chicken, shredded

salt and freshly ground black pepper

PEANUT DRESSING

15g peanuts

juice and grated zest of 1 lime

2 tsp sesame oil

1 tsp runny honey

1 tbsp chopped mint, plus extra leaves to garnish

1 tbsp chopped basil, plus extra leaves to garnish

1 First make the dressing. Put the peanuts in a dry frying pan and toast them gently until golden. Let them cool slightly, then chop them roughly. Put the peanuts and all the other ingredients for the dressing into a small bowl and add a tablespoon of cold water. Season with salt and pepper and mix everything together.

2 Cook the buckwheat noodles in a large pan of simmering water for about 5 minutes or according to the packet instructions. As soon as the time is up, add the mangetout, beans and radishes to the pan, then immediately remove the pan from the heat and drain everything well.

3 Tip the noodle and vegetable mixture into a serving bowl, then add the slices of mango and the chicken.

4 Add the dressing and mix everything together well, then taste and check the seasoning. Scatter over a few extra leaves of mint and basil before you tuck in.

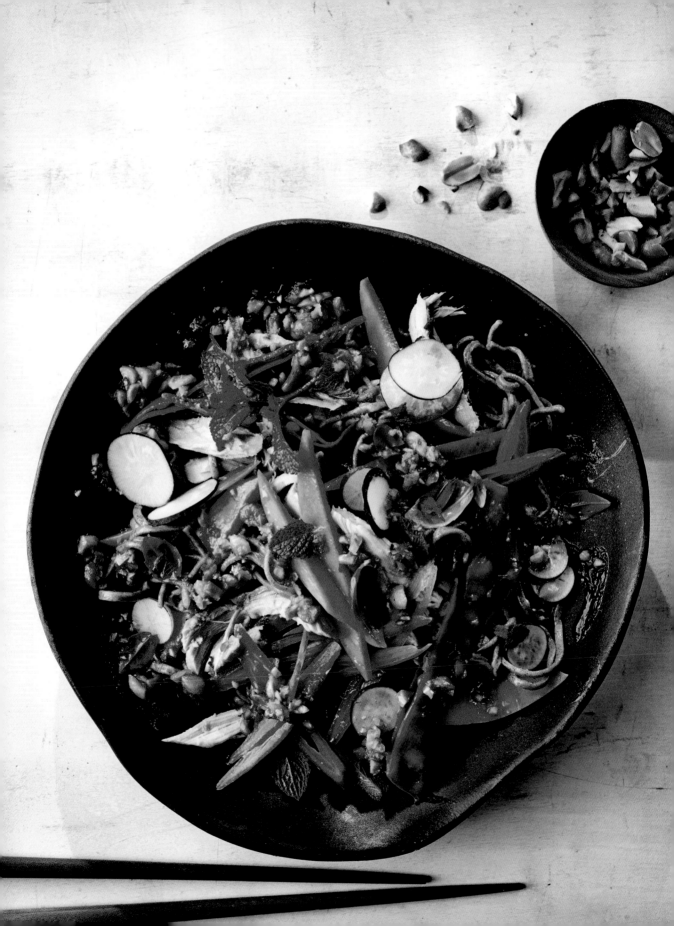

≈ GRILLED SALMON SALAD ≈

Salmon is my number one choice for fish; it's filling, tastes good and it's rich in vitamins and good fats so just right for a healthy meal. This is a great way to enjoy it.

SERVES 2

474 CALORIES PER SERVING

2 x 150g salmon fillets

pinch of paprika

100g sprouting or tenderstem broccoli

50g fresh or frozen peas

1 little gem lettuce, sliced into wedges

50g cucumber, peeled and finely sliced

50g watercress

salt and freshly ground black pepper

DRESSING

1 shallot, finely chopped

1 tsp white wine vinegar

1½ tbsp extra virgin olive oil

juice and zest of ¼ lemon

2 tbsp plain yoghurt

1 Preheat the grill. Sprinkle the salmon fillets with the paprika, then season them with salt and pepper. Grill the salmon for about 10 minutes until cooked through, then set it aside.

2 Meanwhile, start on the dressing. Put the chopped shallot in a bowl with the vinegar. Season it with salt, set it aside for 5 minutes, then strain away the vinegar – this helps to soften the sharp taste of the shallot.

3 Bring a small pan of water to the boil and add the broccoli. Cook it for 3 minutes, then add the peas and continue to cook for 2 minutes more. Drain well.

4 Put the lettuce, cucumber and watercress in a large bowl and add the steamed broccoli and peas. To finish the dressing, add the oil, lemon juice and zest to the chopped shallot and whisk everything together. Spoon half the dressing over the salad, then stir the yoghurt into the remaining dressing.

5 Divide the salad between 2 plates, top with the salmon and serve with the creamy yoghurt dressing to drizzle on top.

TOM'S TIP

If you're planning on making the salmon kedgeree (see p. 30) in the next 2 days, you can cook the salmon fillet for that recipe at the same time as this. Let it cool, then store it in a sealable container in the fridge until needed.

≈

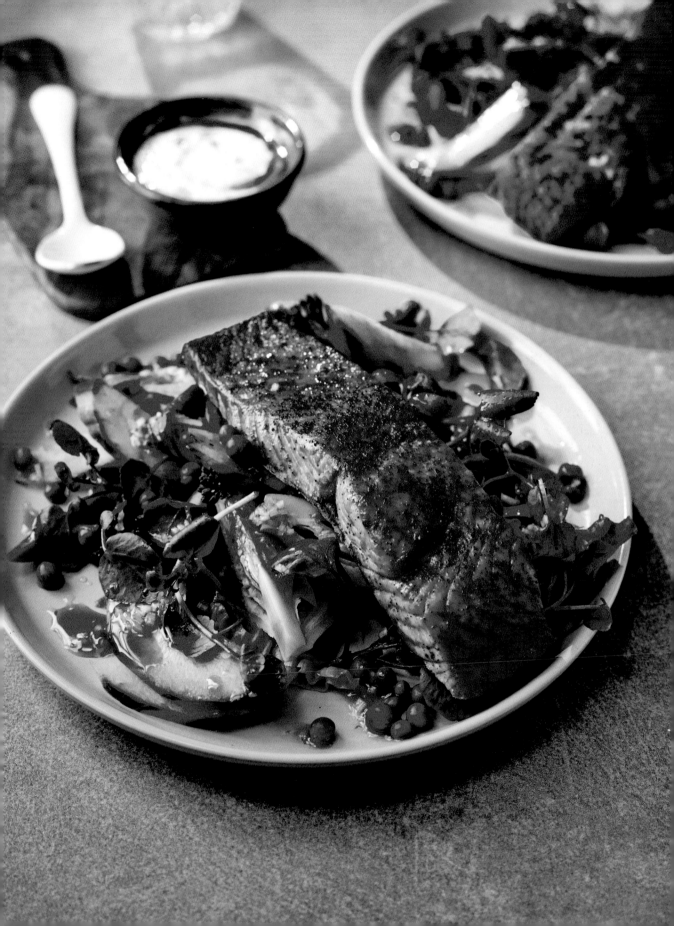

≈ TUNA AND BEAN SALAD ≈

Grilling the vegetables before adding them to the salad may seem like extra work, but I promise you it really is worth it. The grilling softens and sweetens the veg and brings lots of amazing flavour. You can serve this salad on individual lettuce leaves or just pile it on to a bed of shredded lettuce instead.

SERVES 2

269 CALORIES PER SERVING

1 small orange or yellow pepper, halved and deseeded

60g cherry tomatoes (about 6), halved

2 spring onions

115g cannellini beans from a can, drained well

2 tbsp freshly chopped basil and chives, plus a little extra to garnish

150g good-quality tuna (jarred tuna is best), drained of any oil

1 tbsp reserved oil from the tuna or use 1 tbsp extra virgin olive oil

1 little gem lettuce, leaves separated

½ lemon, cut into 2 wedges

salt and freshly ground black pepper

1 Preheat the grill. Put the pepper on a baking tray with the cherry tomatoes and spring onions. Cook until the cherry tomatoes have softened and the spring onions are starting to turn golden – this should take about 8 minutes. Remove the tomatoes and onions from the grill and set them aside.

2 If the skin of the pepper hasn't completely blackened and blistered, continue to grill it until it has. Then put the blackened pepper into a bowl, cover it with a saucepan lid or plate and leave it for 5 minutes to allow the skin to steam away from the flesh.

3 Remove and discard the pepper skin and stalk, then chop the flesh roughly and put it in a bowl. Chop the spring onions and add them and the tomatoes to the bowl. Mix in the beans, herbs, tuna and oil.

4 Arrange the lettuce leaves on 2 plates and spoon the tuna and bean mixture on top of them. Sprinkle with the remaining herbs, then season and serve with lemon wedges to squeeze over the top.

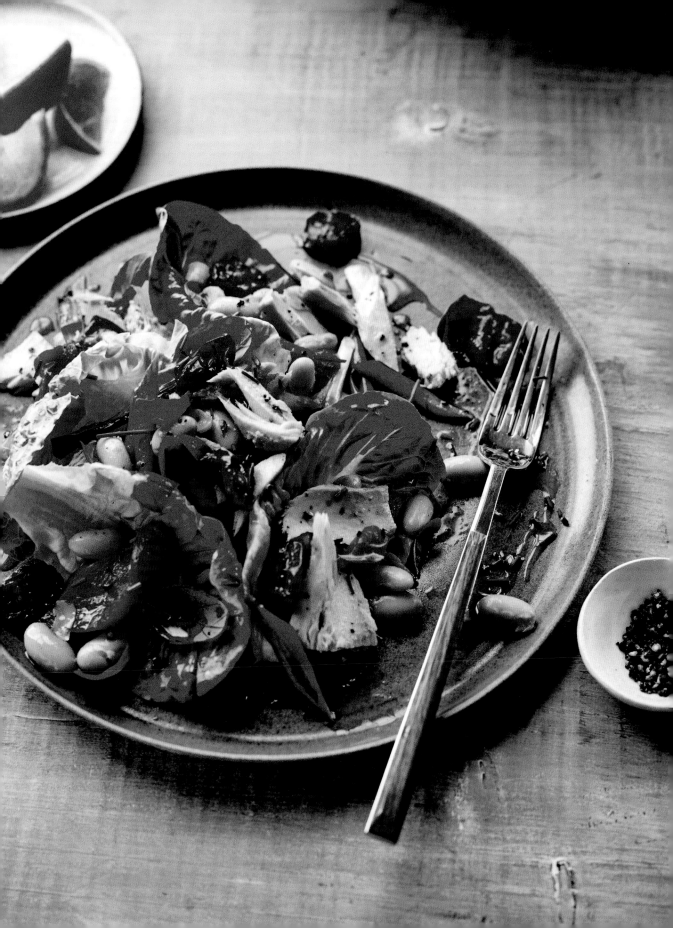

~ BLACK BEAN STEW ~

A cross between a soup and a stew, this recipe packs a punch with the protein-rich beans, a pinch of spice and a topping of pepper, ricotta and avocado. The beans do need to be soaked, but once that's done they're cooked in less than an hour. This stew is so good it's worth making enough for four portions and freezing half if you're not eating it all right away.

MAKES 4 SERVING

181 CALORIES PER SERVING

2 tsp olive oil

½ red onion, chopped

2 celery sticks, chopped

1 tsp fajita spice mix

a couple of thyme sprigs, plus extra to garnish

1 garlic clove, chopped

150g dried black beans, soaked in a bowl of cold water for at least 4 hours, and drained

700ml hot vegetable stock

salt and freshly ground black pepper

TO SERVE

½ red, green or yellow pepper

30g ricotta

½ avocado, flesh chopped

1 Heat the oil in a saucepan and add the onion and celery. Stir in 2 tablespoons of cold water, then season and put a lid on the pan. Cook over a low heat for 10 minutes until the onion starts to soften.

2 Stir in the spice mix, thyme and garlic and continue to cook for 1–2 minutes. Stir in the drained beans and hot stock. Cover the pan again and bring to a simmer, then turn the heat down low and cook for 40–50 minutes until the beans are soft.

3 About 15 minutes before the beans are ready, preheat the grill. Put the pepper half on a heatproof baking tray and grill it until it's blackened and blistered. Put the pepper in a bowl, cover it with a pan lid and leave it to steam for 5 minutes. Peel off the skin, then finely slice the pepper flesh.

4 Take out the thyme sprig, allowing the leaves to fall away into the stew. Discard the sprig. Season the stew well.

5 Serve the stew in bowls and top each bowlful with pepper, ricotta and avocado. Garnish with a few sprigs of thyme. If you want to freeze some of the stew, put it into a sealable container and set it aside to cool before putting in the freezer.

≈ TOM'S TIP

You can freeze this stew for up to three months. I've learned that the best way to defrost it is to leave it overnight in a cool kitchen. When you're ready to eat, reheat the stew in a pan until piping hot before serving.

≈

~ POACHED EGG SALAD ~

Not sure what to make for lunch? I'm sure you'll like this tasty combination of eggs, potatoes and salad, which makes for a fresh and satisfying meal. Non-pareille capers are the tiny ones – they have the best flavour.

SERVES 2

307 CALORIES PER SERVING

175g new potatoes, cut in half if large

100g green beans, trimmed and cut in half

1 slice of sourdough bread (about 40g), whizzed into breadcrumbs

1 tsp olive oil

½ butter or cos lettuce, leaves separated and rinsed

75g baby plum or cherry tomatoes, halved

¼ cucumber, peeled, halved and seeds removed, then finely sliced

1 tsp non-pareille capers

2 large eggs

salt and freshly ground black pepper

DRESSING

1 tbsp extra virgin olive oil

2 tsp red wine vinegar

1 tbsp freshly chopped parsley

1 Bring a small saucepan of water to the boil and cook the new potatoes for about 15 minutes until they're tender. Add the green beans for the last 3 minutes of the cooking time.

2 In a bowl, whisk together the ingredients for the dressing and season well. Drain the vegetables, then tip them back into the pan and add half the dressing. Season with salt and pepper.

3 Put the breadcrumbs in a frying pan and stir in the oil. Cook the breadcrumbs over a medium heat for 3–5 minutes until they're golden, then season with salt and pepper.

4 Divide the lettuce between 2 plates, then add the tomatoes, cucumber and capers.

5 Crack each egg into a small cup or glass. Bring a medium saucepan of water to the boil and use a spoon to swirl the middle. With the water just simmering, drop in the eggs – 1 to each side of the pan – and poach them for 3 minutes. Lift the eggs out with a slotted spoon and drain on kitchen paper.

6 Spoon the potatoes and green beans over the top of the salad, then put a poached egg on top. Scatter over the toasted crumbs and drizzle the remaining dressing on top, then serve.

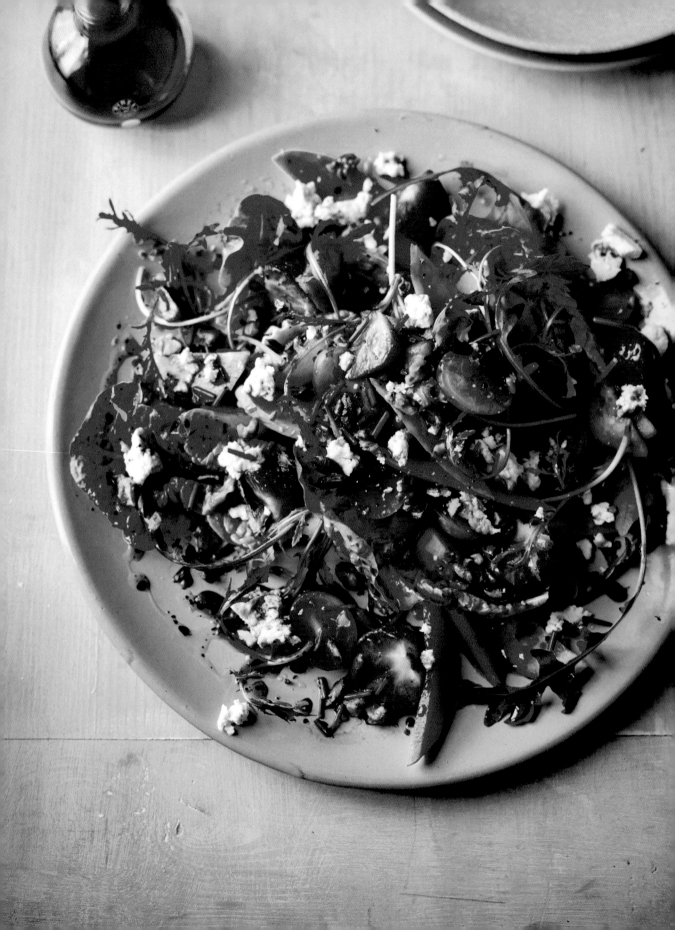

≈ TOM'S SAVOURY FRUIT SALAD ≈

Check out my savoury fruit dish, which is incredibly quick and super healthy. This is great on a really hot day when you don't feel like eating very much but you want something simple and refreshing. I've discovered that the flavours are best if everything is at room temperature when you start – not fridge-cold.

SERVES 2

408 CALORIES PER SERVING

25g walnuts, chopped

10g pumpkin seeds

1 little gem lettuce, leaves separated

¼ cucumber, peeled, halved and deseeded, then finely sliced

½ ripe mango, finely sliced

100g strawberries, hulled and halved

100g green seedless grapes, halved

2 tbsp freshly chopped chives

100g feta cheese, crumbled

small handful of rocket

salt and freshly ground black pepper

DRESSING

1½ tbsp olive oil

1 tsp balsamic vinegar

1 Toast the walnuts and pumpkin seeds in a dry pan for a few moments until golden, then set them aside.

2 Put the little gem leaves in a large bowl or on a serving plate and arrange the cucumber, mango, strawberries and grapes evenly over the top.

3 Scatter over the chives, feta, walnuts, pumpkin seeds and rocket.

4 For the dressing, whisk together the oil and vinegar, then season well. Drizzle the dressing over the salad and serve.

≈ SUMMER SALAD ≈

I've discovered that quinoa has twice the protein of pasta and is a great source of fibre, vitamins and minerals so it's a fantastic alternative to pasta and rice. You can vary this lovely summery salad according to what's available – use asparagus or runner beans, for example, instead of green beans. It keeps well in a sealable container in the fridge so you could always make double quantities and save some for lunch the next day. It's also perfect with some leftover roast chicken.

SERVES 2

268 CALORIES PER SERVING

½ small red onion, finely chopped

1 tbsp red wine vinegar

15g hazelnuts

80g quinoa

75g green beans, trimmed and chopped

½ fennel, finely chopped

½ red pepper, deseeded and finely chopped

2 tbsp freshly chopped herbs such as chives and mint

1 tbsp extra virgin olive oil

juice of ½ lemon

salt and freshly ground black pepper

1 Put the red onion in a large salad bowl and pour the vinegar over the top. Season with a pinch of salt and set the onion aside to marinate – this takes away any harshness in the flavour. Toast the hazelnuts in a dry frying pan for a few minutes, then chop them and set them aside.

2 Put the quinoa in a pan and cover with 225ml of water. Put a lid on the pan and bring the water to the boil. Turn the heat down low and simmer for 15 minutes until the quinoa has absorbed all the liquid and is cooked through and tender.

3 Add the green beans, fennel and pepper to the pan for the last 4 minutes of cooking to steam them until just tender.

4 Drain the red onion and return it to the salad bowl. Stir in the quinoa, vegetables, herbs, oil and lemon juice. Mix well and season with salt and pepper.

5 Divide the salad between 2 bowls, scatter over the toasted hazelnuts, then serve.

TOM'S TIP
To make this more substantial, add 125g of drained chickpeas in step 4.
≈

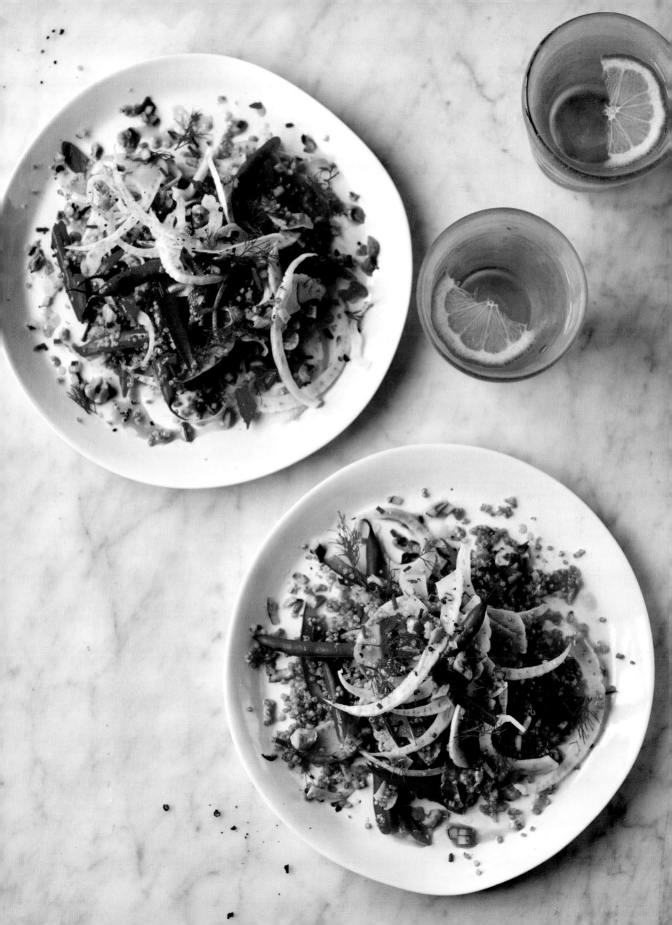

≈ THE NO-BREAD WRAP ≈
WITH TOMATO, FETA AND ROCKET

Do you love a bread wrap? Try this protein-packed alternative, which will keep you full until dinnertime. What you do is make a couple of extra-large, super-skinny omelettes, then spoon in your favourite filling and roll them up. Simple!

SERVES 2

259 CALORIES PER SERVING

75g cherry or baby plum tomatoes, halved

75g feta cheese, chopped

25g rocket, chopped, plus a little extra to serve

small sprig of basil, chopped

1 tsp red wine or balsamic vinegar

1 tsp olive oil

3 large eggs, beaten

salt and freshly ground black pepper

1 Put the tomatoes, feta, rocket and basil into a bowl and toss everything together. Season well, then sprinkle over the vinegar.

2 Heat the oil in a 22–24cm frying pan over a medium heat. Season the beaten eggs and pour half the mixture into the pan, swirling it around so it comes up the sides of the pan. Use a spoon to drag some of the sides to the middle of the pan, then allow the unset runny parts to run into the holes. Continue to do this until the omelette is cooked, then slide it on to a board.

3 Use the rest of the egg mixture to make a second omelette in the same way and slide that on to the board too.

4 Spoon some filling on to both omelettes. Don't overfill them or they will be difficult to roll up neatly. Roll the omelettes up and serve them with any leftover filling on the side.

VARIATIONS

TUNA, RED ONION AND COURGETTE FILLING

251 CALORIES PER SERVING

Mix 100g of good-quality tuna with a quarter of a red onion, chopped, a teaspoon of red wine vinegar and a grated courgette. Add a tablespoon of chopped parsley and season with salt and pepper. Make and fill the omelette as before.

ASIAN-STYLE SALAD FILLING

228 CALORIES PER SERVING

Mix 50g of bean sprouts and 50g of finely shredded white cabbage in a bowl and add half a red pepper, finely sliced, and a grated carrot. Add half a teaspoon of sesame oil, 2 teaspoons of soy sauce and a tablespoon of chopped coriander and mix well. Make and fill the omelette as before.

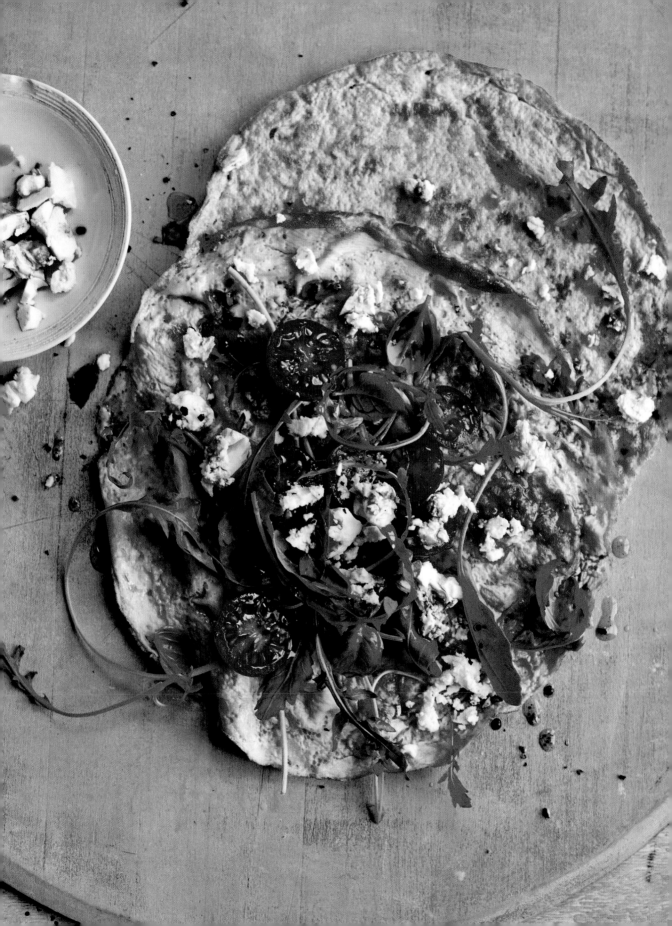

QUICK AND EASY
~ SALAD BOXES ~

Are you a fan of salad boxes? Try these mix-and-match recipes, so you can plan a week of lunches by just combining them with other fresh veg. These are lunchtime winners and can be kept in sealable containers in the fridge for up to four days.

EACH RECIPE MAKES ENOUGH FOR 4 SERVINGS

SOME SALAD BOX IDEAS

Cauli rice, white bean patties, shredded salad and a roast tomato

Cauli steaks, hummus, roast tomatoes and shredded salad

Feta, chopped avocado, roast tomatoes, carrot and cucumber batons, radish

Hummus, roast tomatoes, feta, avocado and shredded lettuce

EXTRAS TO ADD

carrot, grated or cut into ribbons or batons

radishes, halved if large

avocado, flesh chopped

red or white cabbage, finely sliced

cucumber, cut into batons

CAULIFLOWER RICE

52 CALORIES PER SERVING

½ tbsp olive oil

½ small cauliflower (about 165g), whizzed in a blender until finely chopped

1 spring onion, finely chopped

10g pine nuts

10g sultanas

good pinch each of cinnamon and chilli flakes

small handful of freshly chopped parsley

salt and freshly ground black pepper

Heat the oil in a frying pan and add the cauliflower, spring onion, pine nuts, sultanas and spices. Season well and cook for 3–5 minutes, tossing the mixture every now and then until the cauliflower is cooked and starts to turn golden in parts. Stir in the chopped parsley.

CAULIFLOWER STEAKS

26 CALORIES PER SERVING

½ small cauliflower (about 165g), cut into 4 wedges

½ tbsp olive oil

pinch of cayenne pepper

salt and freshly ground black pepper

Preheat the oven to 200°C/180°C Fan/Gas 6. Put the cauliflower in a small roasting tin and drizzle over the oil. Toss to coat, then season with cayenne and the salt and pepper. Roast for 20 minutes until golden and tender.

HUMMUS

137 CALORIES PER SERVING

400g can of chickpeas, drained and rinsed

1 tbsp toasted sesame seeds

2 tbsp extra virgin olive oil

zest and juice of ½ lemon

1 tsp ground cumin

salt and freshly ground black pepper

Whizz all the ingredients in a blender until smooth. Add 1–2 tablespoons of water, season well and whizz again.

ROASTED PLUM TOMATOES

45 CALORIES PER SERVING

4 plum tomatoes, halved or quartered

a little olive oil

salt and freshly ground black pepper

Preheat the oven to 200°C/180°C Fan/Gas 6. Put the tomatoes in a small roasting tin and drizzle over the oil. Toss to coat them all in the oil, then season well. Roast for 20 minutes until golden and tender.

MARINATED FETA

73 CALORIES PER SERVING

100g feta cheese

½ tsp coriander seeds, crushed

good pinch of chilli flakes

1½ tsp olive oil

salt and freshly ground black pepper

Put the feta into a small container and sprinkle over the coriander seeds and chilli. Season well then drizzle the oil over the top.

WHITE BEAN PATTIES

163 CALORIES PER SERVING

25g flaked almonds

2 slices of wholemeal bread

400g can of cannellini beans, drained

small handful of parsley, chopped

2 spring onions, roughly chopped

small handful of fresh coriander, chopped

1 tsp ground cumin

1 tsp ground coriander

a good pinch of hot chilli powder

1–2 tsp olive oil

salt and freshly ground black pepper

1 Toast the almonds in a dry frying pan until golden, then remove the pan from the heat and set the almonds aside.

2 Whizz the bread in a blender or food processor to make crumbs. Add the remaining ingredients, except the oil, season well and whizz again to make a smooth mixture.

3 Divide the mixture into 12 evenly sized pieces and shape them into little round patties or barrel shapes. They don't need to be too neat.

4 Heat a little oil in a frying pan and fry the patties for about 30 seconds on each side until golden – it's best to fry the patties in batches so you don't overcrowd the pan. Set each batch aside as it is cooked.

TOM'S TIP

For a change, try flavouring the feta with some freshly chopped chives or parsley instead of the spices.

LUNCHTIME LIFE HACKS
≈ MAKE THE MOST OF YOUR ≈ LUNCH BREAK

When you're really busy, taking a break in the middle of the day can seem like a waste of time. Lots of us are tempted just to grab a sandwich while checking emails or to skip lunch altogether and work on, but this really doesn't help. We all need time to recharge, so here are my ideas for making the most of your break.

GIVE YOURSELF SOME TIME OUT
Taking a break, even if it's just 15 minutes, has been proved to help you maintain concentration and energy levels throughout the day.

STEP AWAY FROM YOUR DESK
Getting some fresh air can do wonders for your mind and your spirit. Lunchtime, before you've eaten, is also a great time for a workout.

MAKE YOUR ERRANDS EXERCISE-FRIENDLY
If you can't avoid doing errands at lunchtime, make the most of it. Power-walk your way through them and this will revitalise you.

FIND LUNCH BUDDIES
One of the best ways to avoid overeating and keep to a healthy diet is to eat with like-minded people who put an emphasis on good food and nutrition.

GET ORGANISED
Take the opportunity to make a to-do list and look back at what you've achieved in the morning. Feeling like you're in control will free up mental energy and reduce your stress levels.

GIVE YOURSELF TIME OUT, EVEN IF IT'S JUST 15 MINUTES

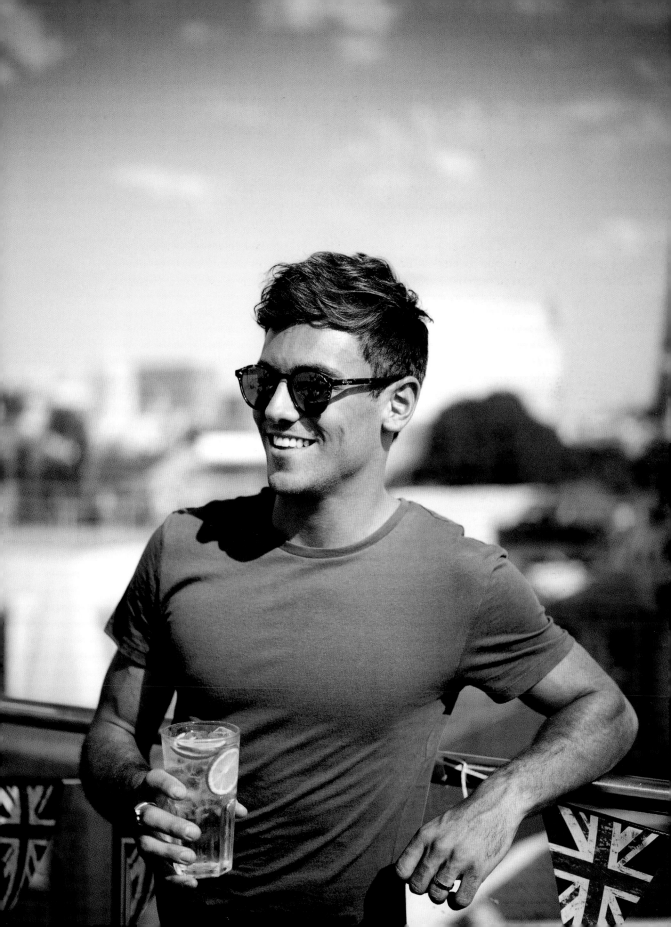

LUNCHTIME LIFE HACKS
≋ STAYING FOCUSED ≋

I often find it can be really hard to keep my attention on the task in hand. And in our hectic world with so much going on all around us, it's tougher than ever. But I know that staying focused is vital for achieving my goals and I've learned some tips that have helped me improve my concentration. I hope they can help you be more productive in every aspect of your life.

FOCUS ON WHAT YOU CAN CONTROL

You only have control over yourself and your own actions and attitudes. You don't have any control over wider outcomes – and thinking about them just creates unnecessary anxiety. Focus on what you're doing and you're more likely to achieve a positive result.

GET RID OF OBVIOUS DISTRACTIONS

None of us likes to be parted from our phones or tablets but if you're doing something important, set your phone aside until you've done what you want to do.

STAY RELAXED

When you're feeling stressed or you're finding it hard to concentrate, think about your breathing. Regulating your breathing not only calms down your circulatory system but will also bring you a feeling of peace so you can focus on the task in hand.

CUT YOUR GOALS DOWN

If you're tackling a task that seems impossible large and difficult, cut it down into manageable chunks and you will find it easier to cope.

LISTEN TO MUSIC

I find listening to music relaxes my mind, hones my concentration and drowns out distractions.

REGULATING YOUR BREATHING CALMS YOU AND BRINGS A FEELING OF PEACE

LUNCHTIME LIFE HACKS
≈ HOW TO BOOST YOUR ENERGY ≈

Like lots of people I'm usually at my best in the morning, then after lunch or in the early afternoon I can start to run out of steam. I've learned how to give my energy levels a boost so I can keep going and make the most of my day. Here are some simple tips that have helped me and might help you too.

DRINK WATER

Water is the main source of energy in the body and I always carry a bottle of water around with me. Don't wait until you feel thirsty to grab a drink of water because you'll already be dehydrated and thirst is a sign that your energy levels are depleted. Always choose water over fruit juices and other drinks – if you get bored, add a slice of lemon or cucumber to your water.

AVOID SNACK FOODS

We all know how easy it is to reach for the biscuit tin when you feel you need an energy boost but don't! Keep away from temptation and keep some healthy snacks, such as a handful of nuts or some of my power balls (see p. 168), to hand.

TAKE A BREAK

As soon as you feel a bit tired and sluggish, walk for ten minutes, preferably outdoors. If you're really pushed for time, even a five-minute stroll around the block will boost your energy levels

STRETCH

If you can't get outside, do some simple and rejuvenating stretches like shoulder rolls. These will get the blood flowing and fight feelings of tiredness

GRAB A COFFEE

Caffeine can be a great pick-me-up – but don't have too much of it. Simple black coffee is low-calorie, cheap and easily available. You'll get energy fast because there's no milk or added fats, so your body will metabolise the coffee more quickly.

IF YOU FEEL TIRED AND SLUGGISH, WALK
FOR TEN MINUTES, PREFERABLY OUTDOORS

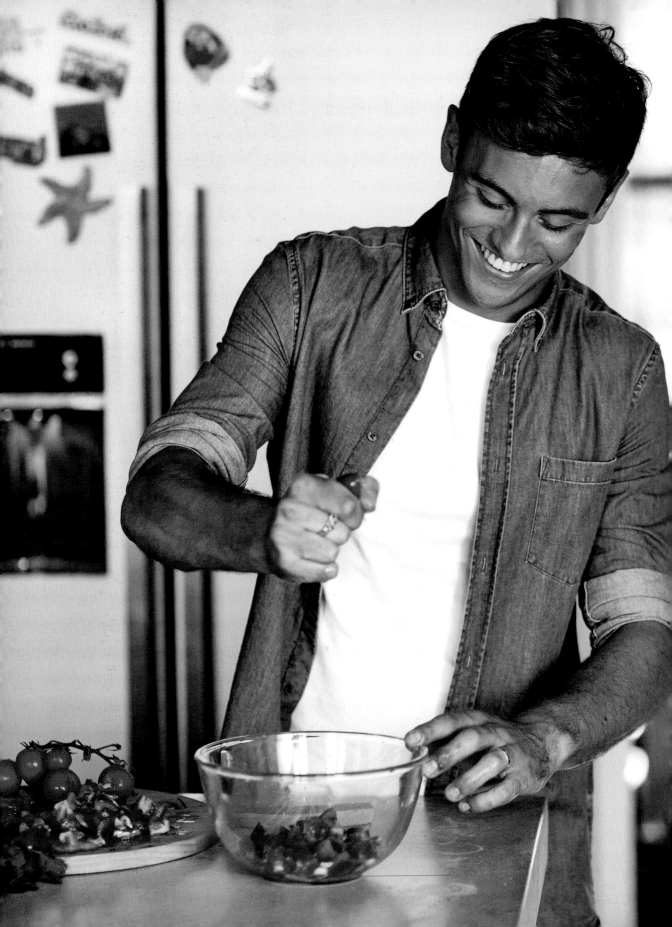

QUICK SUPPERS

≈ BAKED EGGS IN PEPPERS ≈

I love eggs and this is a great way of cooking them. I find that leaving the stems on the peppers when halving and coring them helps to hold the eggs as the pepper roasts and softens. And if you have wobbly pepper halves, level them off by slicing a very thin piece off each base so they sit more steadily in the dish.

SERVES 2

257 CALORIES PER SERVING

2 peppers, halved through the stalk and deseeded

4 anchovies, drained of oil

small handful of rocket or parsley leaves

4 medium eggs

150g green beans, trimmed

25g watercress, washed

1 little gem lettuce, cut into wedges

1 tsp extra virgin olive oil

1 tsp red wine vinegar

2 tsp capers

salt and freshly ground black pepper

1 Preheat the oven to 200°C/180°C Fan/ Gas 6. Put the peppers in an ovenproof dish and place an anchovy and some rocket or parsley into each half.

2 Crack an egg into each pepper half, then season with salt and pepper. Make sure the peppers are sitting steadily in the dish or the liquid white may run out before it has a chance to set. If you prefer, you could wedge the peppers into 4 small individual dishes.

3 Transfer the peppers to the oven and bake them for about 20 minutes until the eggs are nicely set.

4 While the peppers are cooking, bring a small pan of water to the boil. Add the green beans and cook them for 3–4 minutes until tender. Drain them well, then put them in a bowl with the watercress and lettuce. Dress the salad with oil and vinegar and season with salt and pepper.

5 When the peppers are ready, sprinkle a few capers over each half and serve with the salad.

≈
TOM'S TIP
You can also make these with the home-made pesto on p. 106. Spoon the pesto into the base of each pepper half in place of the anchovies and rocket or parsley. Then continue the recipe as above.

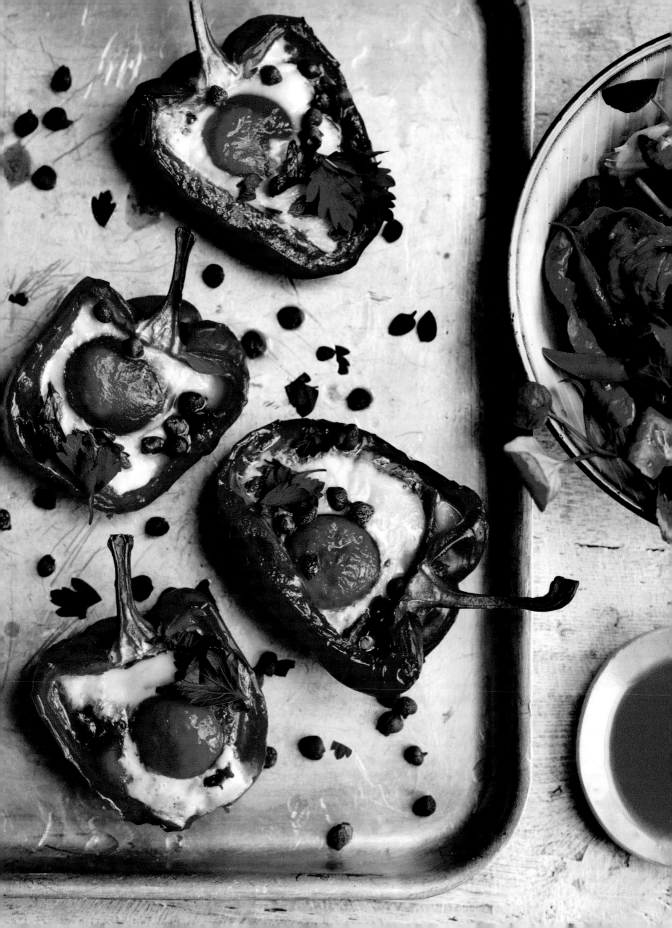

≈ VEGETARIAN PAD THAI ≈

Tofu or bean curd is an excellent source of amino acids, calcium, iron and other micronutrients so really useful for vegetarians. This veggie version of the classic is slightly healthier than the usual, which is often packed with palm sugar. In this recipe, there's just a little sugar to balance the hot chilli and sour tamarind. Serve sprinkled with chopped, toasted nuts, coriander and fresh bean sprouts.

SERVES 2

400 CALORIES PER SERVING

2 tbsp good-quality tamarind paste

35ml hot vegetable stock

2 tsp soy sauce

1 tsp chilli flakes

2 tsp light brown soft sugar

10g peanuts, chopped

1 tsp coconut oil

1 shallot, roughly chopped

2 garlic cloves, roughly chopped

75g mangetout or sugar snap peas, finely sliced lengthways

½ red pepper, deseeded and finely sliced

75g baby corn, halved

1 carrot, cut into strips with a Y peeler

100g rice noodles

small handful of fresh coriander, stems chopped

75g bean sprouts

175g (about ½ pack) silken tofu, roughly chopped

1 Mix the tamarind paste, stock, soy sauce, chilli flakes and sugar in a small bowl and set aside. Toast the peanuts in a dry frying pan for a few minutes, then set them aside.

2 Heat the oil in a wok and add the shallot and garlic and cook for 1–2 minutes. Add the mangetout or sugar snap peas, red pepper, baby corn and carrot strips, then 2 tablespoons of water. Stir-fry the vegetables over a medium heat for 4–6 minutes until they are just tender.

3 Meanwhile, prepare the rice noodles, cooking them until just tender (not soft). Drain them well.

4 Add all but about a tablespoon of the tamarind mixture to the vegetables, along with the noodles, chopped coriander stems and half the bean sprouts. Toss everything together, then divide between 2 bowls. Spoon the remaining bean sprouts and the tofu on top, then drizzle over the rest of the sauce. Scatter some fresh coriander leaves and toasted peanuts on to each bowlful, then serve.

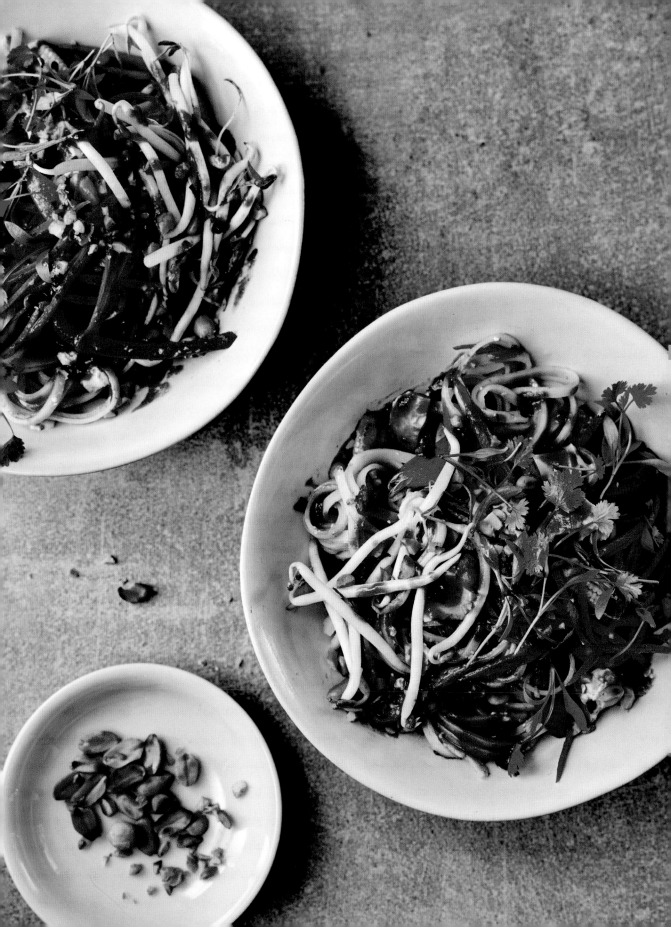

≈ NOODLE SALAD ≈

Easy to make for a packed lunch or a picnic, this combination of wholesome noodles, crunchy veg, prawns and zingy dressing is hard to beat. It's all cooked in one pan so saves on washing up, and it can be made the night before, then stored in the fridge and eaten cold the next day if you like.

SERVES 2

596 CALORIES PER SERVING

2 medium egg noodle nests

2 spring onions, finely sliced

125g white cabbage, shredded

1 large carrot, chopped into thin sticks

4 stems of tenderstem or sprouting broccoli, halved

½ red or orange pepper, finely sliced

100g frozen soya beans

2 radishes, finely sliced

200g shelled raw tiger prawns

a few basil leaves (optional)

DRESSING

1 tbsp sesame oil

2 tbsp soy sauce

juice of 1 orange

½–1 red chilli, finely sliced

1 tsp grated fresh root ginger

1 tsp toasted sesame seeds

salt and ½ tsp ground white pepper

1 Bring a large saucepan of water to the boil. Add the egg noodles and cook them for 3 minutes.

2 Add the spring onions, white cabbage, carrot, broccoli, pepper, soya beans, radishes and prawns to the pan and continue to cook for 1–2 minutes.

3 Meanwhile, make the dressing. Whisk the sesame oil, soy sauce, orange juice, chilli, grated ginger, half the sesame seeds and the seasoning together in a bowl.

4 Drain the noodle mixture, then tip it all back into the pan. Add the dressing and mix well.

5 Serve the salad with the remaining sesame seeds sprinkled over the top and garnish it with basil leaves, if using.

≈ TOM'S TIP

If you make this salad in advance, be extra careful to toss the noodles well with the dressing so they don't stick together too much once cool.

≈

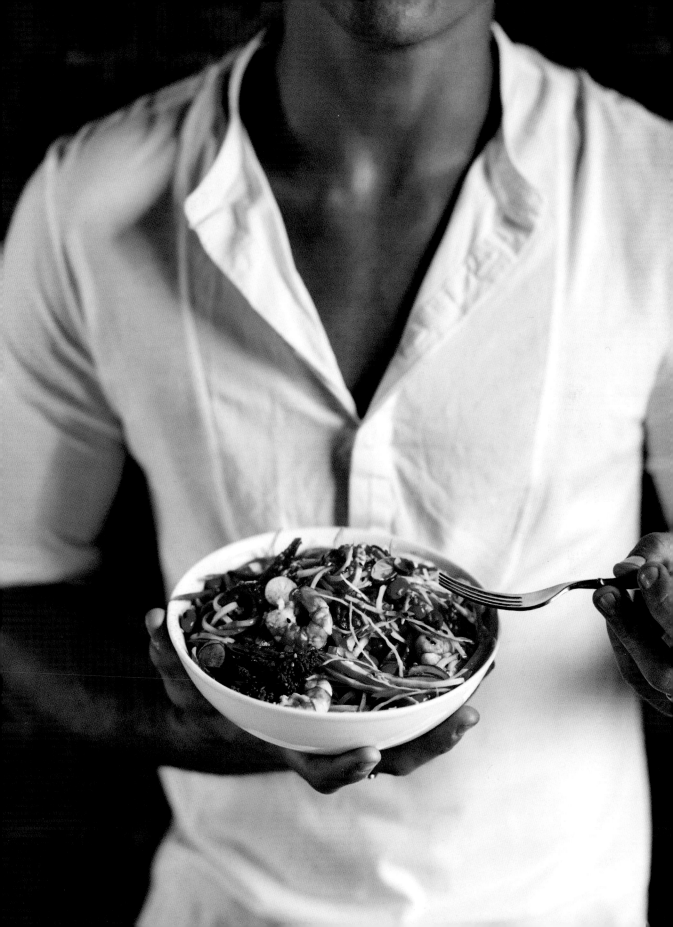

CAULIFLOWER AND EGG
~ HASH BROWNS ~

You'll never miss regular hash browns once you've tried this low-carb, healthy version! It's all cooked in one pan and makes a great brunch or quick supper dish.

SERVES 2

333 CALORIES PER SERVING

1 tbsp olive oil

½ cauliflower including the stalk (about 300g), finely chopped

1 shallot, chopped

2 spring onions, finely sliced

4 medium eggs

small handful of freshly chopped parsley

30g mature Cheddar cheese, grated

good pinch of chilli flakes

salt and freshly ground black pepper

1 Heat the oil in a large frying pan and cook the cauliflower and shallot for 5 minutes. Add the spring onions, season well and continue to cook for another 5 minutes until the cauli is golden brown. Remove the pan from the heat and set it aside to allow the mixture to cool a little.

2 Beat 2 of the eggs in a bowl and stir in the parsley, cheese and chilli flakes. Season well. Stir in the cauliflower mixture, then tip everything into the pan and spread it out to cover the base.

3 Place the pan over a medium heat and make 2 large holes in the mixture with the back of a spoon. Crack an egg into each. Put a lid on the pan and cook over a low to medium heat for 3–4 minutes until the egg whites have set, then serve at once.

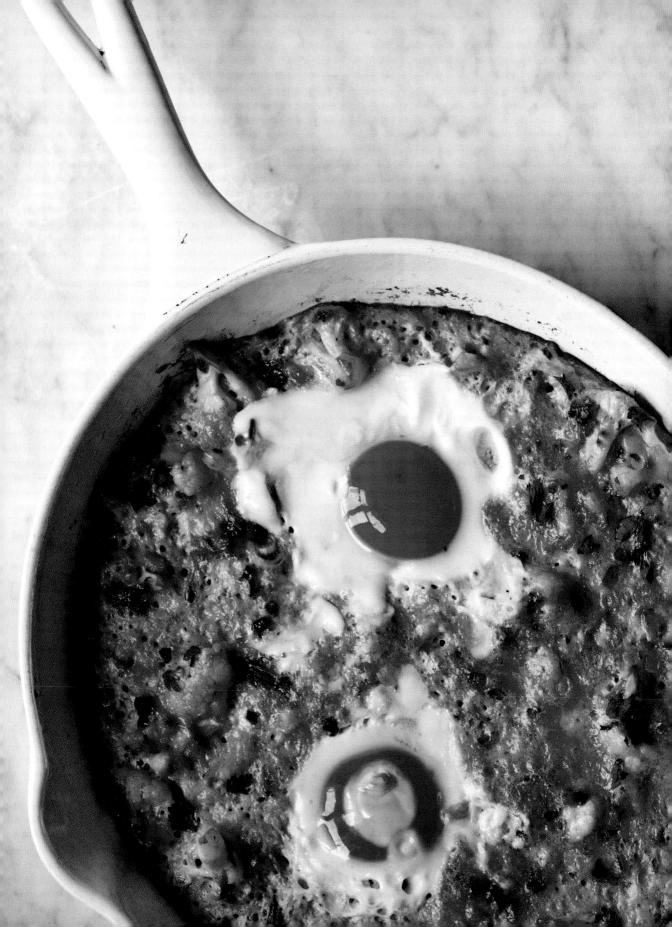

~ CHILLI-SPICED CHICKPEAS ~
WITH SPINACH AND EGGS

Chickpeas are a great food, containing protein, fibre, vitamins and minerals. This recipe is a great post-gym supper – it's ready in minutes and it has a real kick to it from the chilli. I like to add a little drizzle of oil on top too.

SERVES 2

400 CALORIES PER SERVING

1 tbsp olive oil

1 red onion, chopped

1 garlic clove, sliced

½ red chilli, chopped or a good pinch of chilli flakes

200g chopped tomatoes

300ml hot vegetable stock

1 tbsp tomato purée

100g drained and rinsed chickpeas from a can

75g spinach

4 medium eggs

small handful of parsley or fresh coriander, roughly chopped

salt and freshly ground black pepper

1 Heat the oil in a medium saucepan and add the onion. Cook it over a low to medium heat for 10 minutes until it's starting to soften and turn golden. Stir every now and then so that the onion caramelises in the oil. Stir in the garlic and chilli and season well, then cook for 1 minute.

2 Add the tomatoes, stock, tomato purée and chickpeas and stir everything together. Simmer over a low to medium heat for 10 minutes, then season again.

3 Stir in the spinach and let it wilt, then make a dip in the mixture with the back of a large spoon and drop in an egg. Do this 3 more times to add the remaining eggs.

4 Cover the pan with a lid and cook over a low heat for 4 minutes until the whites of the eggs have set – the yolks will be set on the outside but just runny on the inside.

5 Sprinkle over the parsley or coriander and serve at once.

TOM'S TIP
I love this with the eggs but you could also serve just the chickpeas and spinach with some flatbread for a light supper.
≈

≈ SPICED SQUASH AND BUTTERBEANS ≈

Another good vegetarian recipe, this simple pan-fried supper is a real winner. The cucumber pickle takes only a few moments to make and the fresh tangy flavour really adds to the dish.

SERVES 2

521 CALORIES PER SERVING

100g brown basmati rice (optional)

1 tbsp coconut oil

1 shallot, chopped

350g butternut squash, chopped

1 tsp cumin seeds, crushed

1 tsp coriander seeds, crushed

1 tsp mustard seeds

1 garlic clove, chopped

1 red chilli, deseeded and chopped

200g plum tomatoes (4–5), quartered or use 200g chopped tomatoes from a can

200ml hot vegetable stock

400g can of butterbeans, drained

2 tbsp Greek yoghurt

small handful of freshly chopped coriander

salt and freshly ground black pepper

CUCUMBER PICKLE

¼ cucumber, peeled, halved, deseeded and finely sliced

25ml white wine vinegar

good pinch each of unrefined caster sugar and salt

pinch of chilli flakes

1 First make the pickle. Put the cucumber, vinegar, sugar, salt and chilli flakes in a bowl and mix well. Set the pickle aside.

2 If you're going to serve this with rice, put the rice in a saucepan and pour over 250ml of just-boiled water. Cover the pan with a lid, bring the water back to the boil, then turn the heat down low and cook the rice according to the packet instructions.

3 Heat the oil in a large wok and add the shallot and squash. Cook for about 5 minutes until the vegetables are starting to soften, tossing them every now and then. Stir in the cumin, coriander and mustard seeds and the garlic and chilli and cook for 1 minute. Season well.

4 Add the tomatoes to the pan, pour over the stock and stir in the butterbeans. Cover the pan and cook for a further 15–20 minutes until the stock has reduced slightly and the squash is tender.

5 Divide the rice, if serving, between 2 plates, then top with the squash stew. Add a spoonful of yoghurt to each portion, sprinkle with fresh coriander and serve with the cucumber pickle.

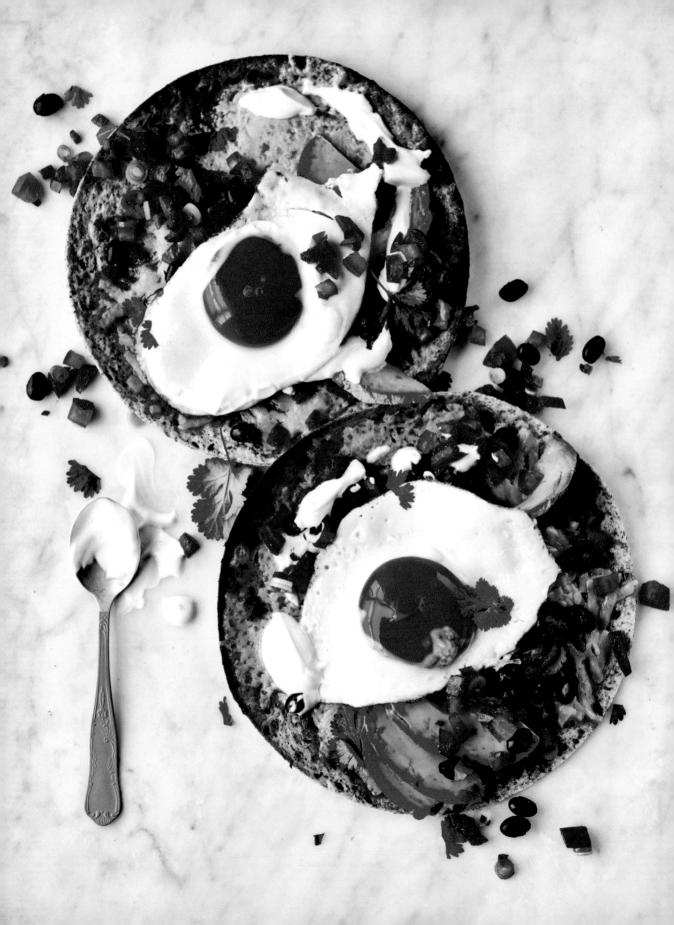

≈ HUEVOS RANCHEROS ≈

This Mexican-inspired dish is one of my all-time favourites. It's very quick
to prepare – while the tortillas are toasting, you can whip up the salsa and cook
the fried eggs. Flavourful and hearty, this also makes a fab breakfast! If you
like your food extra hot, add a whole chilli instead of just half.

SERVES 2

486 CALORIES PER SERVING

2 small wholemeal tortillas

30g mature Cheddar cheese, grated

1 tsp olive oil

2 medium eggs

½ avocado, sliced

2 tsp soured cream

salt and freshly ground black pepper

SALSA

2 spring onions, finely chopped

2 fresh tomatoes, chopped

½ red pepper, deseeded and finely chopped

½–1 red chilli, deseeded and chopped

100g drained black beans (about ½ can drained)

¼ tsp ground coriander

squeeze of lime

1 tbsp freshly chopped parsley or coriander

1 Preheat the grill. Put the tortillas on the grill pan, scatter the cheese evenly over them, then grill until golden.

2 To make the salsa, mix the onions, tomatoes, pepper, chilli, black beans, ground coriander, lime and parsley or coriander in a bowl, then season well.

3 Heat the oil in a small frying pan and add half a tablespoon of water. Bring the water to the boil and allow it to evaporate a little bit, then add the eggs. Cover the pan and cook the eggs until the yolks are just set.

4 Serve the toasted cheese tortilla topped with some bean salsa, slices of avocado and the fried eggs, then dollop the soured cream on top. Serve immediately.

≈ TOM'S TIP

This makes quite a lot of salsa but if
you don't use it all in this dish, it keeps
well in the fridge for up to 3 days,
stored in a sealable container.

≈

≈ SALMON PARCELS ≈

Salmon, sweet potato and other veggies – all gathered into a parcel and steamed in the oven. Job done! Cooking the lemon wedges at the same time makes them deliciously jammy and gets lots of sweet juice out of them. One thing I find – the sweet potato does need to be chopped quite small otherwise it won't cook in the time.

SERVES 2

485 CALORIES PER SERVING

2 tsp olive oil

zest of ½ lemon (cut the zested lemon in half)

½ tsp coriander seeds, roughly crushed

¼ tsp fennel seeds, roughly crushed

1 small courgette, sliced

4 cherry tomatoes, halved

1 small corn on the cob, kernels sliced off

1 small sweet potato (about 165g), cut into 1cm dice

2 x 150g salmon fillets

small handful of coriander, chopped

salt and freshly ground black pepper

1 Cut out 2 large pieces of baking paper (about 38cm square) and set them aside. Preheat the oven to 200°C/180°C Fan/Gas 6.

2 Put the oil, lemon zest and the coriander and fennel seeds in a large bowl, season well and stir. Then add the courgette, tomatoes, corn and sweet potato and toss well to coat everything in the oil.

3 Divide the vegetables between the 2 pieces of paper, placing some in the middle of each one. Top with the salmon, then season with salt and pepper.

4 Take a parcel, bring 2 sides of the paper together and twist the ends to secure, leaving a gap in the centre. Spoon 2 tablespoons of cold water into the gap, then fold the paper over a couple of times to secure it. Repeat with the second parcel, then put them both on a baking tray. Put the wedges of lemon on the baking tray too.

5 Bake the parcels in the oven for 20–25 minutes until the sweet potato is tender. Serve sprinkled with chopped coriander and the cooked lemon wedges to squeeze over the salmon.

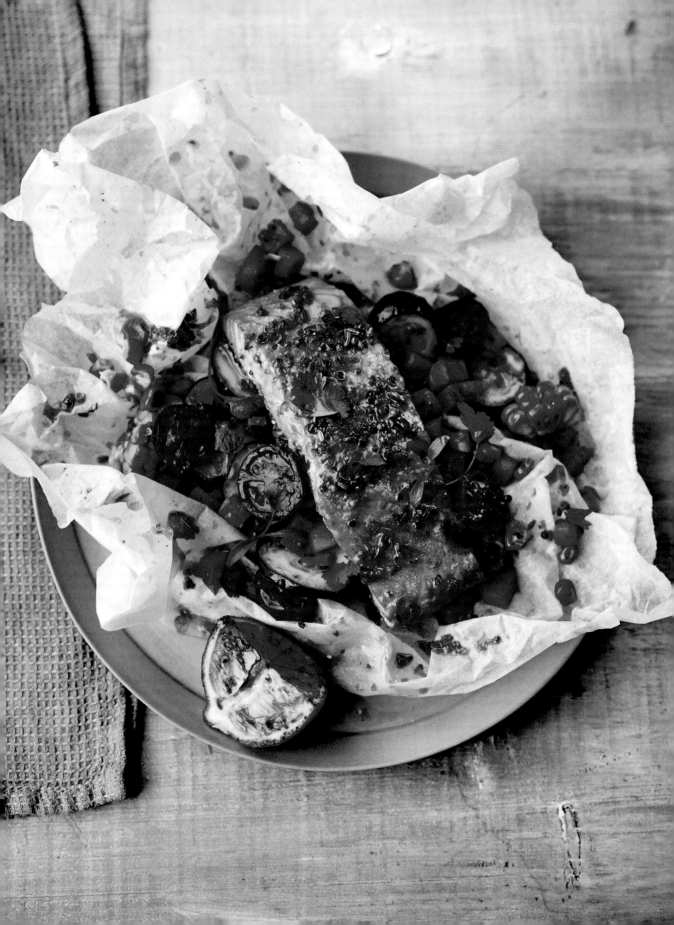

~ COD AND LENTILS ~

I love salmon but I'm also a big fan of white fish, which is another good source of vitamins and minerals. Pancetta adds a salty depth to the lentils and is a good balance for the delicate cod. This might sound like a very simple supper, but it's really satisfying.

SERVES 2

343 CALORIES PER SERVING

80g puy lentils

2 small sprigs of rosemary

2 slices of lemon

2 x 150g cod loins

6 slices of pancetta

1 tbsp olive oil

1 garlic clove, sliced

½–1 red chilli, chopped

100g kale, chopped

100g cherry tomatoes, halved

salt and freshly ground black pepper

1 Put the lentils in a saucepan and cover them with plenty of cold water. Put a lid on the pan and bring the water to the boil, then turn the heat down low and simmer the lentils for 15 minutes until they're just tender but still have a slight bite. Drain well.

2 Put a rosemary sprig and a slice of lemon on to each piece of cod and season with salt and pepper. Then wrap each piece of cod in 3 slices of pancetta.

3 Heat a teaspoon of the oil in a frying pan, add the pancetta-wrapped cod and cook for about 2 minutes until golden. Use tongs to turn the pieces over to brown the other side. Add a tablespoon of water and put a lid on the pan. Turn down the heat and cook for 5 minutes until the cod is cooked through.

4 Heat the remaining oil in a pan and cook the garlic and chilli for 1 minute. Add the kale, cherry tomatoes and 75ml of just-boiled water and cook for about 5 minutes until the kale is tender. The tomatoes will be lovely and squishy by this stage, too. Stir in the lentils and season well.

5 Divide the lentil mixture between 2 plates and top with the cod. Spoon over any juices from the pan and serve.

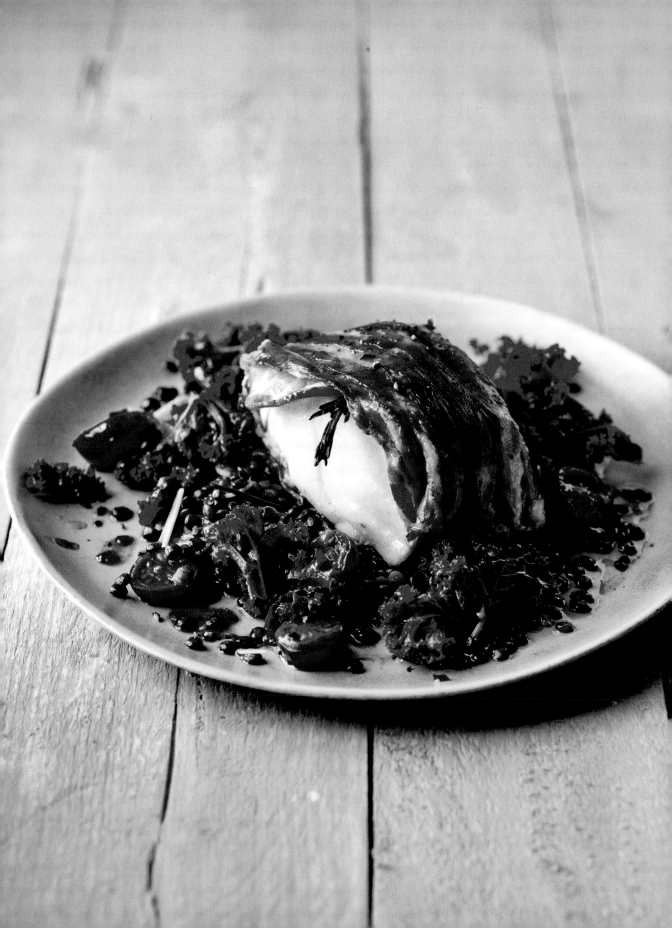

≈ HARISSA PRAWNS ≈

Hot, aromatic harissa puts a mouth-watering spin on this speedy midweek supper – and if you'd like it even spicier, add half a chopped chilli. You could also make this with wholegrain rice or quinoa for a change from couscous.

SERVES 2

677 CALORIES PER SERVING

1 tsp olive oil

2 spring onions

½ red pepper, deseeded and chopped

½ fennel bulb, chopped

½ medium courgette, chopped

1 garlic clove, chopped

1 tsp ground coriander

1 tsp harissa paste

200g chopped tomatoes

150ml hot vegetable or chicken stock

225g raw peeled king prawns

100g wholewheat couscous

zest of ½ lemon

small handful of fresh coriander or parsley, stalks finely chopped

10g whole almonds, chopped

2 tbsp Greek yoghurt

salt and freshly ground black pepper

1 Heat the oil in a saucepan, add the spring onions, pepper, fennel and courgette, then cook over a medium heat for 5 minutes. Stir in the garlic, coriander and harissa and cook for a further 1–2 minutes.

2 Stir in the tomatoes and stock and season well. Bring the sauce to a simmer, then continue to cook for about 5 minutes until the vegetables are just tender and the sauce has thickened slightly. Turn the heat down to low, stir in the prawns and cook them for about 3 minutes longer, until they've all turned pink.

3 Meanwhile, prepare the couscous. Put it in a heatproof bowl, add the lemon zest and chopped herb stalks, then season with salt and pepper. Pour over 125ml of just-boiled water, cover the bowl (a pan lid,

baking tray or even a plate will do) and set it aside for 5 minutes while the couscous absorbs all the liquid. Fluff it up with a fork. Toast the almonds in a dry pan for a few moments, then set them aside.

4 Serve the couscous, spoon the saucy prawns on top and scatter over the almonds and remaining herbs. Add a spoonful of yoghurt on the side.

TOM'S TIP

Frozen raw prawns are fine for this so it's great to have some in the freezer, ready to take out and thaw overnight in the fridge.

≈

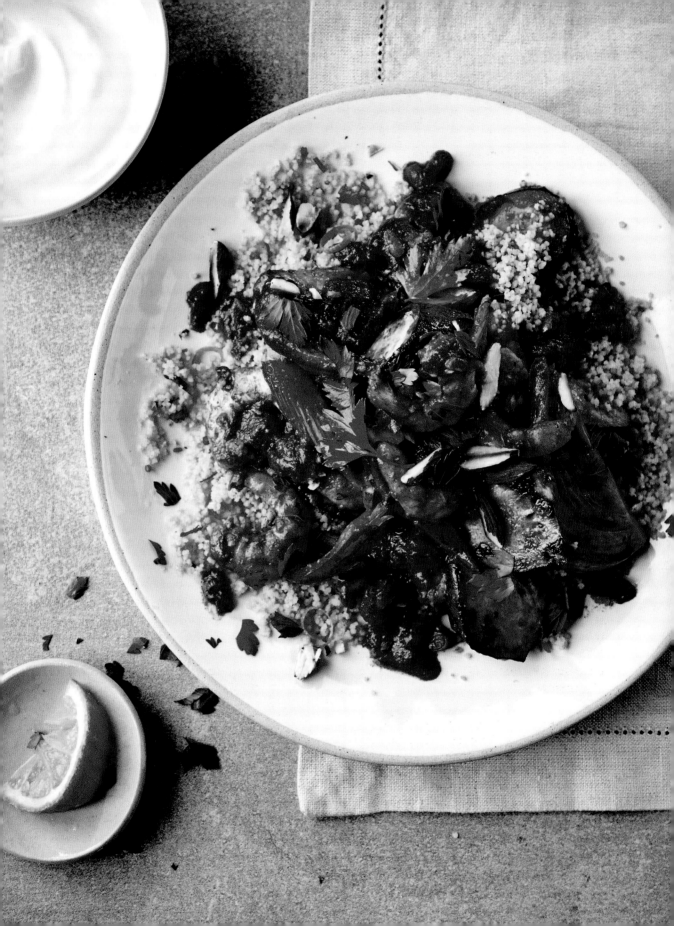

≈ QUICK STIR-FRIED PRAWNS ≈
WITH PAK CHOI

Fancy something special for supper? Try this super-quick and tasty dish
that will rival anything from your local Chinese takeaway! Good-quality
prawns are key for the best flavour.

SERVES 2

373 CALORIES PER SERVING

2 tsp coconut or sesame oil

2 garlic cloves, sliced

10g fresh root ginger, finely
sliced

1 tsp Chinese five-spice powder

300g raw peeled tiger prawns

2 pak choi, cut in half

100g flat rice noodles

2 tsp soy sauce

1 tsp sesame seeds, toasted

1 Heat the oil in a large frying pan or wok,
then add the garlic, ginger and five-spice
powder. Cook for 1 minute, then add the
prawns and cook for another minute,
tossing once.

2 Add the pak choi and a tablespoon of
water, then cover the pan with a lid.
Turn the heat down low and cook until
the pak choi is tender and the prawns
have turned pink.

3 Meanwhile, cook the rice noodles
according to the packet instructions.

4 Drain the noodles and divide them
between 2 bowls. Stir the soy sauce into
the prawn mixture and spoon the mixture
over the noodles, drizzling any sauce from
the pan over too. Sprinkle the sesame seeds
on top and serve at once.

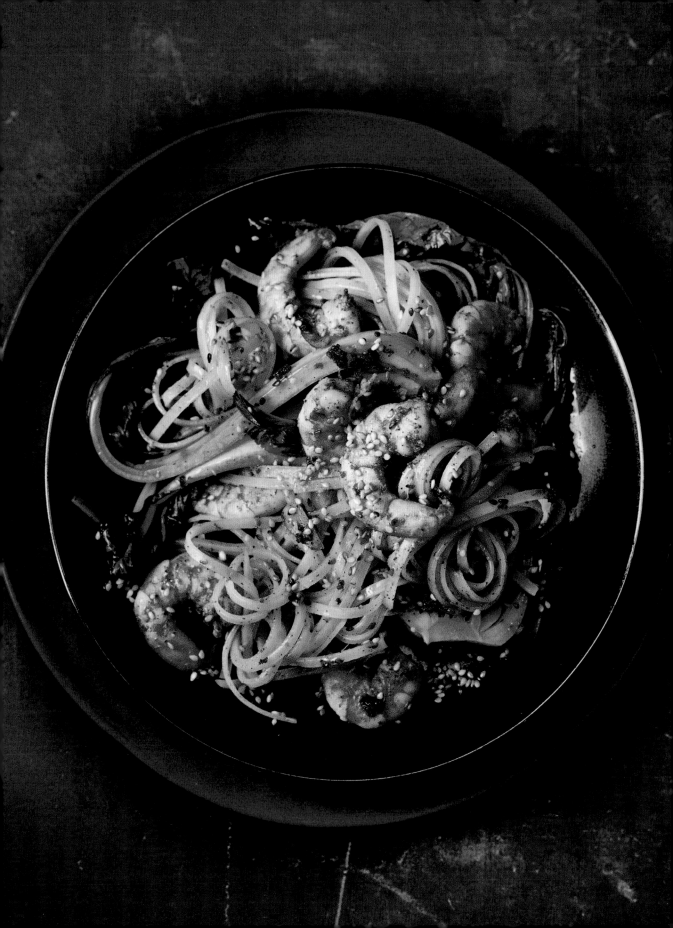

≈ FAJITA-STUFFED CHICKEN ≈

If you're a huge fan of fajitas like me, this is a cool way of serving chicken, with all the flavourings of a fajita. One tip I've learned is that some fajita seasonings contain sugar so check the label and find one without – it really doesn't need it.

SERVES 2

333 CALORIES PER SERVING

2 tsp olive oil

2 spring onions, chopped

¼ red pepper, deseeded and finely chopped

1 garlic clove, crushed

1 tsp fajita seasoning

1 tsp dried thyme

1 tbsp cream cheese

10g mature Cheddar cheese, grated

2 x 125–150g skinless, boneless chicken breasts

200ml hot chicken stock

salt and black pepper

BEAN SALAD

1 corn on the cob, kernels sliced off

100g green beans, finely chopped

100g mixed beans from a can, drained

1 tbsp freshly chopped coriander, plus extra to garnish

1 Heat 1 teaspoon of the oil in a frying pan and cook the spring onions and pepper over a medium heat for 5 minutes. Season well and stir in the garlic, fajita seasoning and thyme and cook for another minute. Tip it all into a bowl and allow to cool, then stir in the cream cheese and grated Cheddar.

2 Lay a chicken breast on a board. Slice horizontally through the thickest part of the meat, but don't cut it right through to the edge. Open the chicken breast out like a book. If there's a flap at the back of the chicken piece, there's no need to cut it, just open that out too. Repeat with the other chicken breast.

3 Put half the filling on one of the pieces of chicken, then fold it over again and secure with a couple of cocktail sticks. Repeat with the rest of the stuffing and the other piece of chicken.

4 Heat the remaining olive oil in a frying pan and cook the chicken on each side until golden. Pour the stock into the pan and cover with a lid. Cook for about 20 minutes until the chicken is cooked through and no pink juices remain.

5 Bring a saucepan of water to the boil, add the corn and green beans, then bring the water back to the boil. Drain the corn and beans in a colander and quickly cool them under cold running water to refresh and stop the cooking process. Put the corn, green beans, drained mixed beans and chopped coriander into a bowl. Season well.

6 When the chicken is cooked, transfer the pieces to a board and cut them into slices. Pour any sauce left in the pan into the bean salad and stir it in, then divide it between 2 plates. Top with the chicken, garnish with chopped coriander and serve.

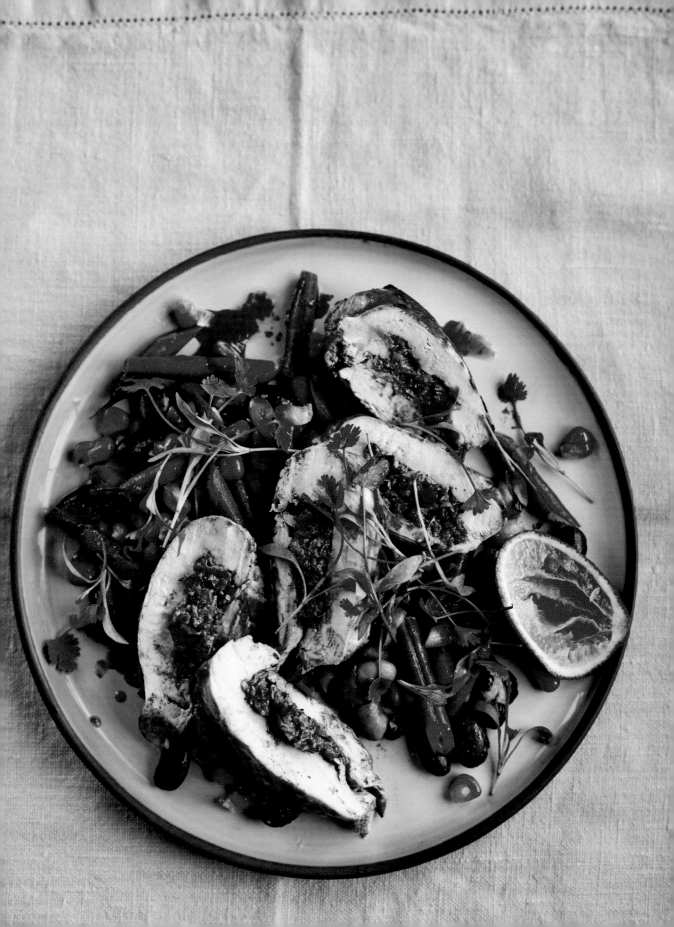

≈ CHICKEN, MOZZARELLA AND PESTO ≈
FILO PARCELS

When you need something a bit more filling than a salad for dinner, try
this easy recipe. I'm a massive fan of the combination of mozzarella, sun-dried
tomatoes and pesto, and these crunchy little parcels are amazing.

SERVES 2

671 CALORIES PER SERVING

1 tbsp olive oil

8 large basil leaves,
finely chopped

1 tsp pine nuts

225g skinless, boneless chicken
breast or thigh meat, chopped

3 sun-dried tomatoes,
finely chopped

125g mozzarella, chopped

4 rectangular sheets
(about 170g) of filo pastry

20g butter, melted

salt and freshly ground
black pepper

1 Preheat the oven to 200°C/180°C Fan/
Gas 6. Preheat a baking tray.

2 Put the oil, basil and pine nuts in a
mortar and grind them with a pestle
until smooth. If you don't have a pestle
and mortar, just chop the basil and nuts
as finely as you can. Season well.

3 Put the chicken, tomatoes and mozzarella
into a bowl and add the pesto. Season well
and stir everything together.

4 Lay the 4 sheets of filo pastry on a board
then cut them in half to make 2 squares
(each piled with 4 sheets). Set one pile aside
and with the other pile, twist each square
around slightly to make a star outline.

5 Spoon half the mixture on to one of
the piles of pastry. Brush a little melted
butter around the base, then gather up the
outsides and scrunch them together to make
a large money-bag shape. Brush half of the
remaining butter over the top. Do the same
with the remaining ingredients and filo.

6 Transfer the parcels to the preheated
baking tray and bake them in the oven
for about 25 minutes until golden. Serve
with some green vegetables or salad.

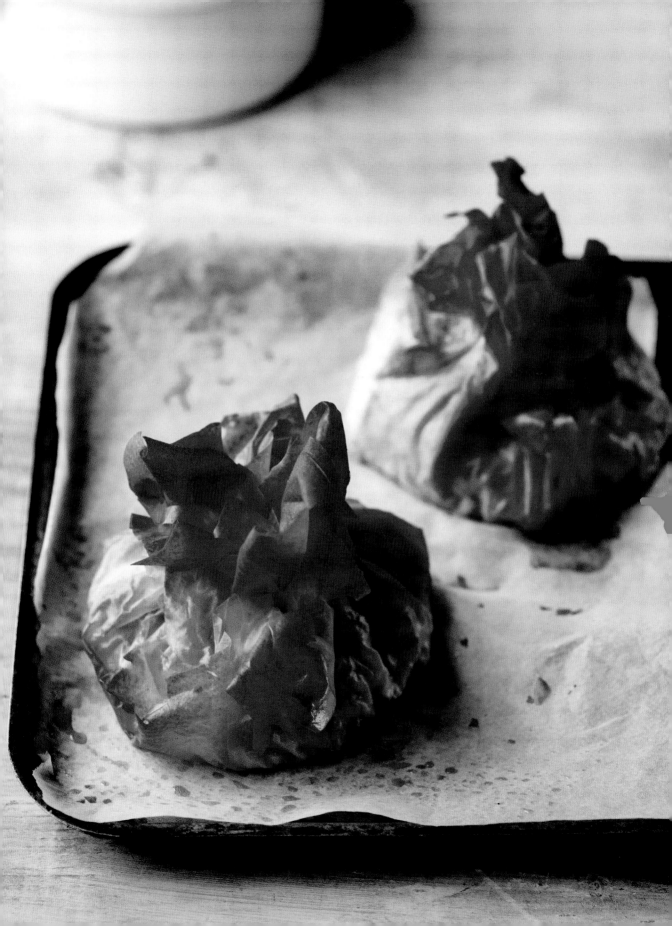

~CHICKEN CURRY~
WITH TOMATO AND COCONUT

This curry dish is surprisingly straightforward to make, tastes amazing and it's a fraction of the calories of a takeaway curry. If you want to get ahead with the preparations you can make the spice paste up to a day earlier and keep it in the fridge, then gently reheat it on the hob before using. If you don't like your food very spicy, leave out the chilli powder.

SERVES 2

515 CALORIES PER SERVING

100g brown basmati rice, washed

2 tsp coconut or sunflower oil

½ red onion, chopped

1 fat garlic clove, sliced

10g fresh root ginger, cut into slivers

3 skinless, boneless chicken thighs (about 300g), chopped

2 tomatoes, each cut into 8 wedges or 200g chopped tomatoes from a can

200ml chicken stock

100g frozen peas

25g coconut cream, chopped

handful of coriander, chopped

sea salt and freshly ground black pepper

SPICE PASTE

1 tsp ground cumin

¼ tsp ground turmeric

1 tsp ground coriander

½ tsp chilli powder (optional)

½ tsp ground black pepper

1 tbsp tomato purée

1 Put the rice into a saucepan and cover it with 300ml of cold water. Add a pinch of salt and put a lid on the pan. Bring the water to the boil, then turn the heat down low and simmer the rice until all the water has been absorbed – this will take about 25 minutes. Leave the lid on the pan but turn off the heat and set the rice aside.

2 Mix together all the ingredients for the spice paste.

3 Heat the coconut or sunflower oil in a large frying pan and cook the onion over a medium heat for 3–4 minutes until it's starting to turn golden. Add the garlic and ginger and cook for 1 minute. Season well.

4 Stir in the spice paste and cook for 2–3 minutes. Add 2 tablespoons of water and stir until it has been absorbed. Do this a few more times until the paste looks like a sauce. Add the chicken and tomatoes, then brown the chicken in the pan for about 5 minutes, turning it halfway through. Season well.

5 Stir in the stock, cover the saucepan with a lid and bring the stock to a simmer. Reduce the heat to low and cook for 10 minutes. Add the peas and the coconut cream, check the seasoning and simmer for another 2–3 minutes.

6 Divide the rice between 2 bowls, spoon over the chicken curry and garnish with the coriander.

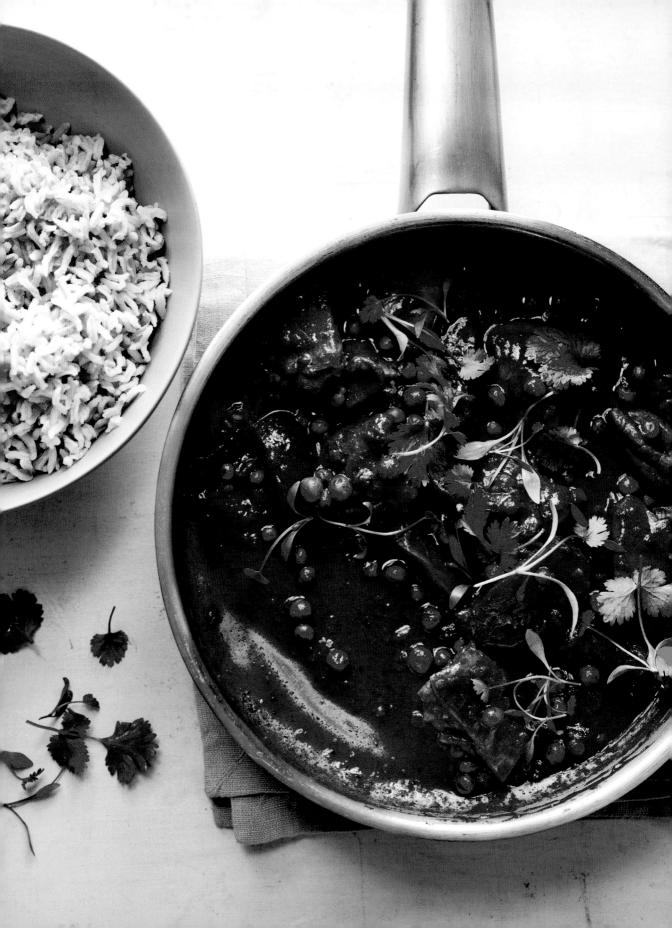

≈ FLAT-IRON CHICKEN ≈
WITH BROCCOLI

Chicken breast and broccoli is a great meal to have after a workout and an excellent source of protein to help repair muscles. Bashing out the chicken gives you a bit of an extra workout too! I'm sure this will become a big favourite so I've suggested a variation with a different sauce.

SERVES 2

300 CALORIES PER SERVING

2 x 150g skinless, boneless chicken breasts

1 tsp olive oil

sea salt and freshly ground black pepper

BROCCOLI

300g head of broccoli, cut up into florets, or 300g tenderstem broccoli

8 cherry tomatoes, chopped

20g stoned black olives, chopped

2 tbsp freshly chopped parsley

1 tsp extra virgin olive oil

1 tsp red wine vinegar

½ garlic clove, crushed (optional)

1 Line a large board with cling film and lay a chicken breast on top, smooth-side down. Take a sharp knife and slice horizontally through the thick part of the chicken towards the other side, taking care not to slice all the way through the meat.

2 Open out the chicken breast like a book, then cover it with another sheet of cling film and bash with a rolling pin until it's about 3mm thick all over. Remove the cling film, season the meat well and brush with half the oil. Set the chicken aside on a plate while you do the same with the other piece.

3 Heat a griddle pan until hot and cook the chicken pieces for 4–5 minutes on one side until golden. Turn them over and cook on the other side for a further 3–4 minutes.

4 Meanwhile, bring a pan of water to the boil. Add the broccoli and cook for 2–3 minutes until just tender. Drain the broccoli well and put it back in the pan. Add the tomatoes, olives, parsley, oil, vinegar and garlic, if using. Toss well.

5 Put a chicken piece on each plate, add the broccoli mixture and serve.

CHIMICHURRI CHICKEN AND BROCCOLI
Prepare the chicken breasts as before and sprinkle over a little smoked paprika after seasoning. Cook the broccoli as above until just tender and drain it well. Tip it back into the pan, then add 1½ tablespoons of chimichurri sauce (see p. 144), toss well and serve it with the chicken.

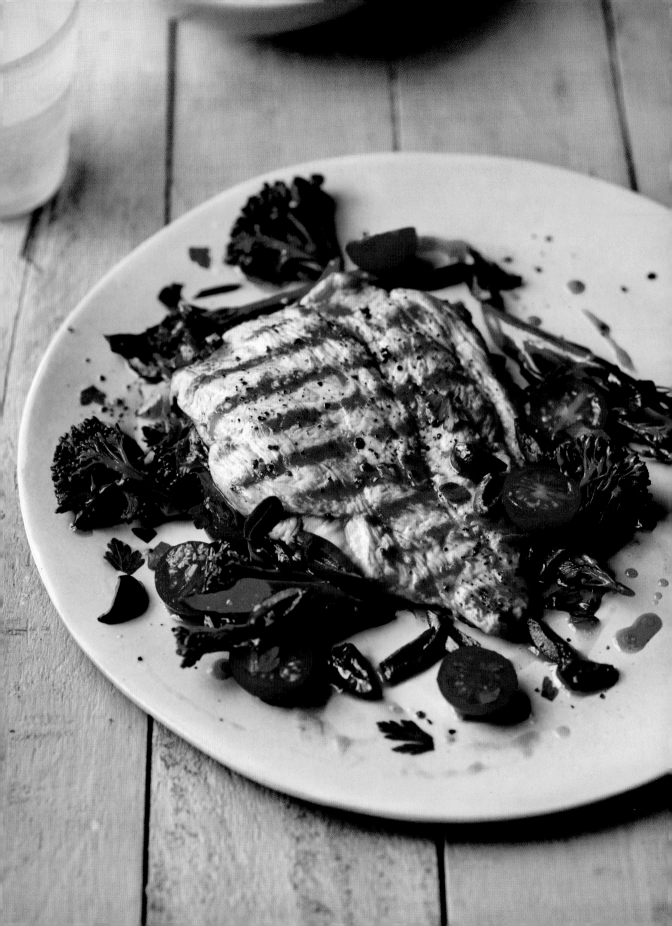

≈ SINGAPORE-STYLE NOODLES ≈
WITH PORK

Here's my version of this classic noodle dish, served with marinated lean pork.
It really is hot so if you're not so keen on very spicy food, start with half a
tablespoon of curry powder and leave out the chilli. It does take a little while to
prepare all the vegetables, but once that's done, this is super quick to cook.

SERVES 2

460 CALORIES PER SERVING

½ tsp turmeric

1 tbsp medium curry powder

½ tsp ground white pepper

1 tsp grated fresh root ginger

½ red chilli, chopped

200g pork tenderloin, trimmed
and sliced into thin slivers

1 tsp coconut oil

2 spring onions, trimmed,
halved and finely sliced into
long strands

1 courgette, spiralised or sliced
into noodles with a Y peeler

1 large carrot, spiralised or sliced
into noodles with a Y peeler

½ red pepper, finely sliced
lengthways into thin strands

1 tbsp peanut and coconut
butter (see p. 172)

100g rice noodles

small handful of coriander

½ lime, cut into wedges

salt and freshly ground
black pepper

1 Put the turmeric, curry powder, ground
white pepper, ginger and chilli into a
large bowl. Add the pork, season with a little
salt and stir everything together. Set the
bowl aside while you prepare the rest of
the ingredients.

2 Heat the oil in a large wok and add
the pork. Cook it over a medium heat
for about 3 minutes, then add the spring
onions, courgette, carrot and pepper. Season
well and continue to cook for 5–6 minutes
more. The mixture will look very dry at first,
but the vegetables will cook down and
moisten the dish as they steam. Stir in the
peanut and coconut butter and a tablespoon
of water and season well.

3 Meanwhile, cook the rice noodles
according to the packet instructions.
Drain well and add the noodles to the
pan with the pork and vegetables. Toss
everything together, then serve in bowls
and top with the coriander. Add some
lime wedges on the side.

≈
TOM'S TIP
If you haven't made the peanut
and coconut butter on p. 172,
just use a tablespoon of regular
peanut butter instead.

≈

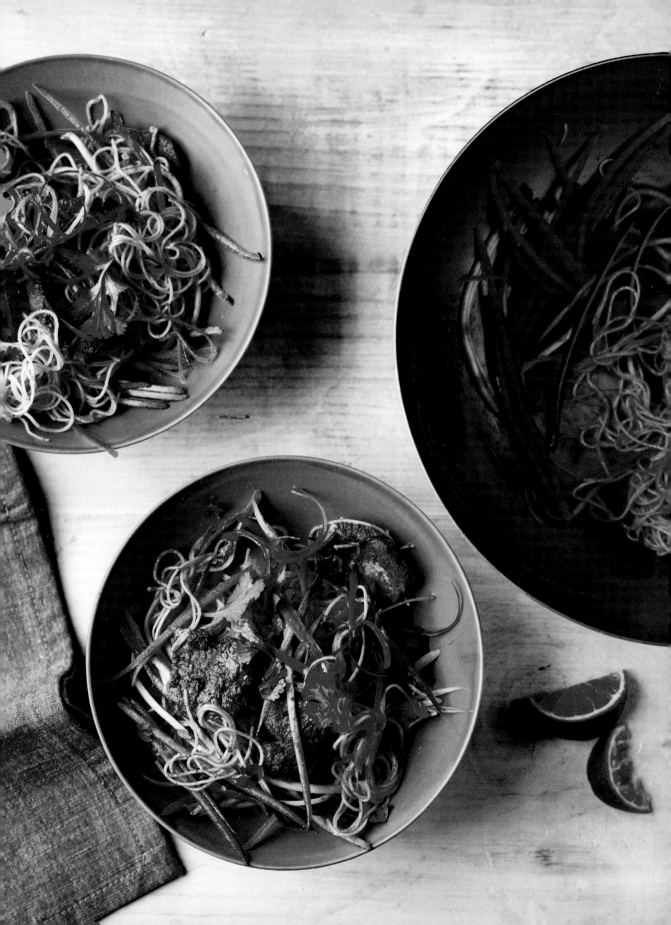

≈ LANCE'S SCOTCH EGGS ≈

This is Lance's healthier take on a Scotch egg. There's no breadcrumb
coating or deep-frying but these are still really good to eat.

SERVES 2

469 CALORIES PER SERVING

2 medium eggs

250g pork or beef mince

1 large shallot, finely chopped

1 large sprig of rosemary,
finely chopped

a little oil

salt and freshly ground
black pepper

1 Bring a small saucepan of water to the boil
and cook the eggs for 8 minutes. Put them
in a bowl of cold water and leave them to
cool, then peel off the shells.

2 Put the mince in a bowl, add the shallot
and rosemary, season and mix well. Wet
your hands and take half the mixture, then
spread it out to a thickness of about half a
centimetre. Season the meat well and place
an egg on top, then wrap the mince around
it, squeezing it at the join to seal the seam.

3 Do the same with the other portion of
mince and egg. Rub a little oil over each
ball and season again.

4 Heat a dry frying pan over a medium
heat until just hot. Fry the balls for 15–20
minutes, turning them frequently until they
are golden brown all over. They are ready
when they feel firm. You can take a peek
inside one to see if the mince is done and
continue to cook if you need to. Serve
with a big crisp salad.

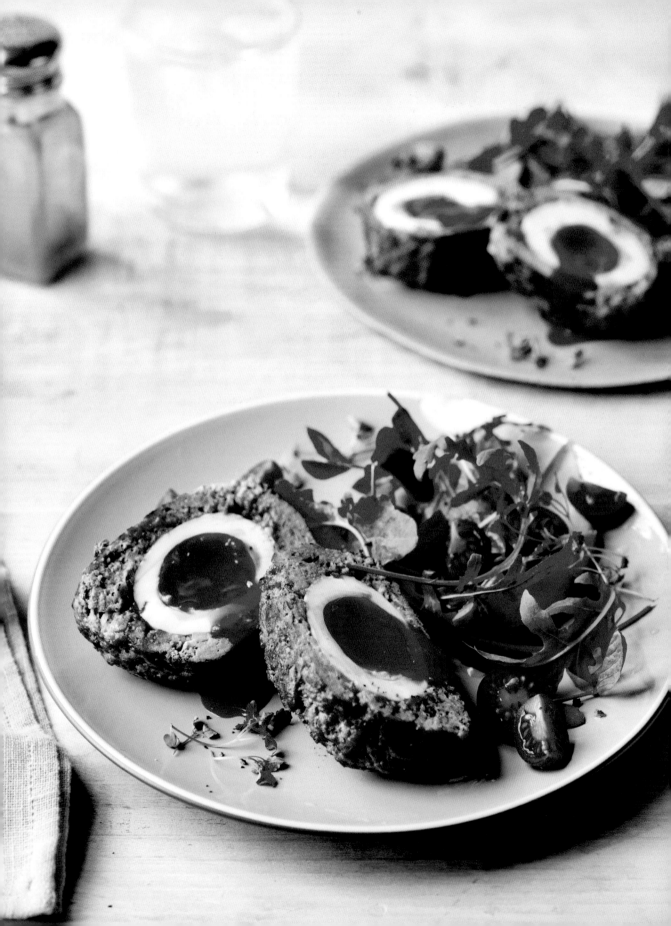

~ GRIDDLED LAMB CHOPS ~
WITH SWEET POTATO MASH

I think this makes a really special supper and it's quick and easy to make. Lamb cutlets have the best flavour and they're trimmed of fat so they're nice and lean. If you can't find them in your supermarket, check out your local butcher – the meat there can often be cheaper and better quality. You need a ridged griddle pan for this recipe – the kind with a handle and sides – which is a really useful piece of kit for grilling meat and fish.

SERVES 2

575 CALORIES PER SERVING

1 tsp olive oil

1 tsp red wine vinegar

1 sprig of rosemary, leaves finely chopped

4 lamb cutlets, trimmed of fat

2 sweet potatoes (about 250g), chopped

125g purple sprouting broccoli or green beans, trimmed

150ml hot chicken stock

5g butter

salt and freshly ground black pepper

1 Put the oil, vinegar and rosemary in a shallow dish and season well. Add the lamb chops and toss them in the mixture, then set them aside to marinate. You can leave them out of the fridge if you're going to be cooking them soon, but if you want to get ahead, you can put the chops in the marinade the day before and store them in a sealable container in the fridge.

2 Put the sweet potatoes in a saucepan and cover them with water. Put a lid on the pan, bring the water to the boil and cook the sweet potatoes for about 12 minutes or until soft. Drain, leaving a couple of tablespoons of water in the pan. Tip the potatoes back into the pan, season and mash them well.

3 Cook the broccoli or beans in a separate pan of boiling water. Drain them well and keep them warm.

4 Heat a griddle pan until hot. Turn the heat to medium, then add the chops to the pan. Cook them for 3–5 minutes on each side.

5 Once the chops are cooked, put them on a plate and keep them warm. Add the stock to the pan and bring it to the boil. Season well and simmer until the stock has reduced by half. Stir in the butter and any juices from the resting lamb to add more flavour.

6 Serve the mash and broccoli or beans, top with the lamb chops and spoon the sauce around them.

≈ VEGETABLE TOTS ≈

A great little vegetable side to serve with steak, sausages, chicken, lamb or fish, these are a real crowd-pleaser. They're lovely hot just out of the oven but also good cold, so they're great for a picnic.

SERVES 2

392 CALORIES PER SERVING

50g oats

125g broccoli

1 spring onion, finely chopped

50g mature Cheddar cheese, grated

25g ground almonds

½ tsp cayenne

1 tsp fresh thyme

2 medium eggs

salt and freshly ground black pepper

1 Preheat the oven to 200°C/180°C Fan/ Gas 6. Line a large baking tray with some baking paper.

2 Whizz the oats in a blender until finely chopped. Break the broccoli into florets and whizz that in the blender too until finely chopped.

3 Put the oats, broccoli, spring onion, cheese, ground almonds, cayenne and thyme in a bowl. Season well and mix everything together.

4 Make a well in the middle, add the eggs and beat them with a fork. Gradually fold in the ingredients until everything is combined and the eggs have been incorporated into the mixture.

5 Scoop up a teaspoonful of the mixture and roll it into a little sausage shape. Place it on the baking tray. Continue until you've used up all the mixture – you should have about 16 tots. If the mixture seems a little sticky, set it aside for 5 minutes while the oats and almonds absorb the egg.

6 Bake the tots in the oven for 20–25 minutes until golden.

TOM'S TIP
Try adding some freshly chopped chilli to these for a spicy kick.
≈

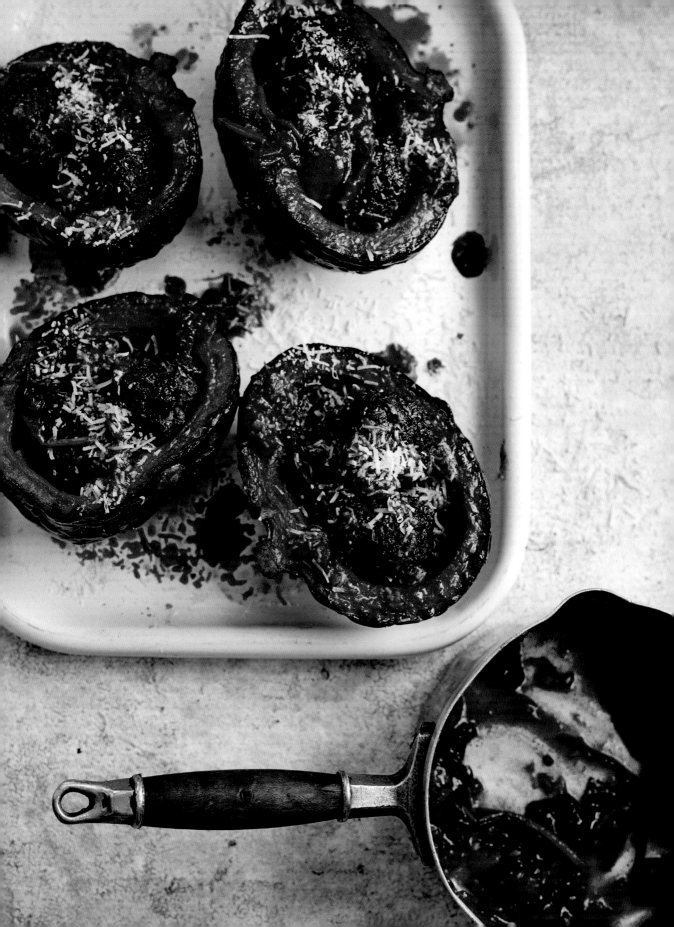

≈ MEATBALL-STUFFED SQUASH ≈
WITH SPINACH SAUCE

There are lots of great flavours in this hearty, tasty dish, which is always a massive hit with Lance and my friends. Acorn squash work well as they are just the right size for the meatballs, but you could use any kind.

SERVES 2

500 CALORIES PER SERVING

2 small squash, such as acorn, (each about 300g), halved and deseeded

1 shallot, peeled

2 tbsp freshly chopped herbs such as parsley, chives, sage and basil

20g whole almonds, chopped

20g stoned black olives

40g Parmesan cheese, grated

250g lean beef mince

salt and freshly ground black pepper

SPINACH SAUCE

1 tsp olive oil

2 garlic cloves, sliced

200g chopped tomatoes (from a can)

200ml hot vegetable stock

100g spinach

1 Preheat the oven to 200°C/180°C Fan/Gas 6. Cut the squash in half and remove the seeds. Put the squash halves in a roasting tin, spoon a tablespoon of water into each half and cook them in the oven for about 30 minutes.

2 Put the shallot, herbs, almonds, olives and half the Parmesan cheese in a small food processor and whizz until finely chopped. Tip everything into a bowl, add the mince and season with salt and black pepper. Mix thoroughly, then divide into 12 rough portions.

3 Shape each portion of the mixture into a ball and drop 3 balls into each squash half. Sprinkle with the remaining cheese. Turn the oven down to 180°C/160°C Fan/Gas 4 and continue to bake the squash for 20–30 minutes until the mince is cooked through.

4 Meanwhile, make the sauce. Heat the oil in a small pan, add the garlic and cook it for 1 minute until it's just starting to turn golden. Add the tomatoes and stock and season well. Cover the pan with a lid and simmer for 15 minutes, then stir in the spinach and allow it to wilt. Serve the sauce with the squash.

EVENING LIFE HACKS
≈ EAT MINDFULLY ≈

You hear a lot now about 'eating mindfully' and at first I wasn't sure what this really meant. In fact, it's very simple. It means paying proper attention to the experience of eating and drinking and to the textures, flavours and smell of food. If you ever find yourself having a meal in front of the television or while catching up with some emails and hardly noticing what's on your plate, it's time to change. Mindful eating plugs us back into our body's cues, so we know when we need to eat and when we've had enough. Here are some ideas to try.

ENJOY EACH BITE
Think about the texture and flavour of each mouthful you eat. How do you feel before and after?

REMOVE DISTRACTIONS
Never eat in front of the television and remove your phone from the table! Did you know that it takes 20 minutes for our brains to register that we are full? That means if you're distracted by other things at mealtimes, it's all too easy to overeat.

RELAX AT MEALTIMES
It's generally accepted that if we eat when we're stressed, the body does not digest food in the same way and cannot derive the same full nutritional value from it as when we're feeling calm. Try to eat at regular times.

THINK ABOUT YOUR FOOD
Thinking about what we're eating can help us to develop a healthier relationship with food and to lose weight. Also, think about your food and where it came from? If you take the time to understand more about the origins of the food you eat, you'll gain a deeper appreciation and this might change your eating habits.

KEEP A FOOD DIARY
Write down everything you eat and why. Did you eat because you were hungry? Or were you tired, bored or stressed? By becoming more aware of our emotional eating triggers and patterns it's easier to adjust them and make healthy changes.

MINDFUL EATING PLUGS US BACK INTO OUR BODY'S CUES SO WE KNOW WHEN WE'VE HAD ENOUGH

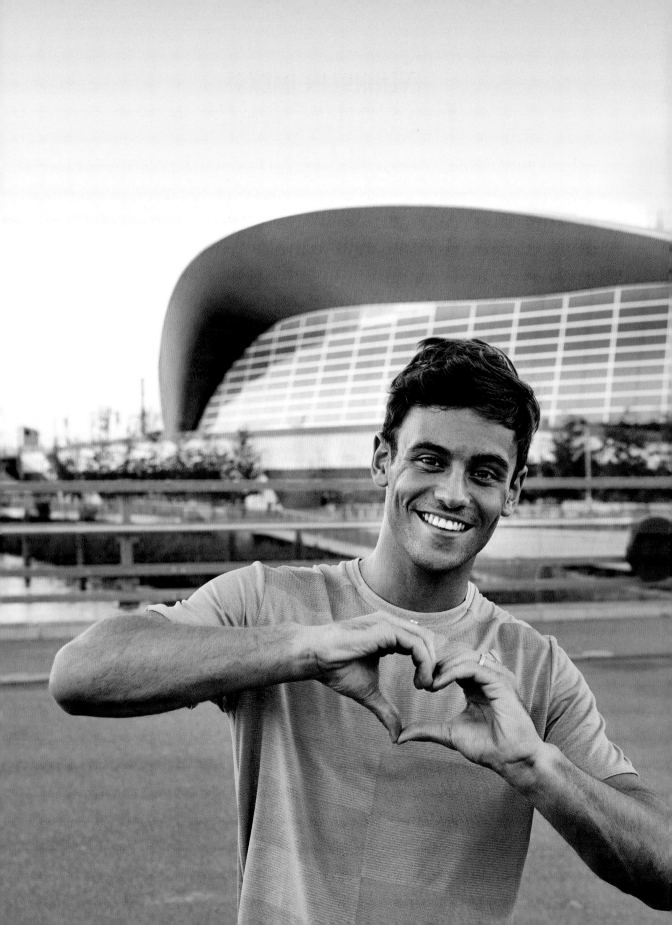

EVENING LIFE HACKS
≋ THE GOOD THINGS ≋
IN LIFE

I'm lucky – I know I am. I do something I love, I have a wonderful partner and a supportive family and I probably don't always appreciate everything as much as I should. We all know we should acknowledge what we feel grateful for more regularly, but it's all too easy to get caught up with what's going wrong in our lives or obsessing about what we don't have.

Research shows that gratitude has powerful effects on physical health, self-worth and personal relationships. People who show their gratitude and appreciation also have stronger immune systems, sleep better and are fitter.

Gratitude and happiness are intertwined and for a good reason. If you want to feel happier, then try to boost your level of gratitude. Regular appreciation for what's around you brings feelings of optimism, whether it's about the big things in life – being healthy or having good friends – or stuff on a smaller scale, like receiving a nice email or enjoying the sun shining.

END YOUR DAY ON A POSITIVE NOTE

One of the simplest ways of practising gratitude is to think about – and write down if you wish – a few things that you are grateful for. The ideal time to do this is in the evening, before you go to sleep.

For me, some days it's as simple as having had a great chat with a friend, or a certain part of my training going well, or thinking about my amazing family.

Even on days that aren't that great, there'll always be something positive you can feel grateful for. This will end your day on a bright and happy note!

REGULAR APPRECIATION FOR WHAT'S AROUND YOU BOOSTS FEELINGS OF OPTIMISM, WHETHER IT'S ABOUT THE BIG THINGS IN LIFE OR STUFF ON A SMALLER SCALE

EVENING LIFE HACKS
≋ MY BEST-EVER SLEEP TIPS ≋

I know that if I don't have enough sleep I'm not at my best the next day. Sleep is such a crucial part of a healthy lifestyle. If you sleep well, you'll wake up feeling refreshed, alert and capable of doing all the things you had planned much more quickly and effectively than if you are sleep deprived. Here are my top tips for getting that perfect night's sleep.

KEEP IT REGULAR
Waking up at the same time and going to bed at the same time will help programme your body to sleep better.

MAKE YOURSELF COMFORTABLE
Keep your bedroom as a rest space, not a workspace – keep screens out of the room. Make sure it's not too hot or too cold and keep it as quiet and dark as possible when it's time to get some shuteye.

RELAX
Take a hot bath, listen to some soothing music or do some meditation before bedtime.

DON'T SMOKE!
Smokers take longer to fall asleep, wake more often and experience more sleep disruption. And that's in addition to the obvious health reasons for giving up.

CUT DOWN ON CAFFEINE
Fizzy drinks and chocolate as well as coffee and tea contain caffeine. Cutting down helps if you struggle to drift off at night.

DON'T OVER INDULGE
Too much food or alcohol, especially late at night just before bedtime, can play havoc with sleep patterns. Alcohol may help you get to sleep initially but will interrupt your sleep later on in the night.

KEEP ACTIVE
Exercising regularly really does help relieve the stress and strains of the day. If you can't do a proper workout, try to fit in some sort of exercise, even just a brisk walk – but not too close to bedtime or it might keep you awake!

MAKE A LIST
If you find yourself worrying about what you have to do tomorrow, get it all out of your head. Make a list of what you have to do the next day, then tell yourself not to think about it any more.

DO SOMETHING!
If you can't sleep, don't lie there worrying about it. Get up and do something you find relaxing until you feel sleepy again, then go back to bed.

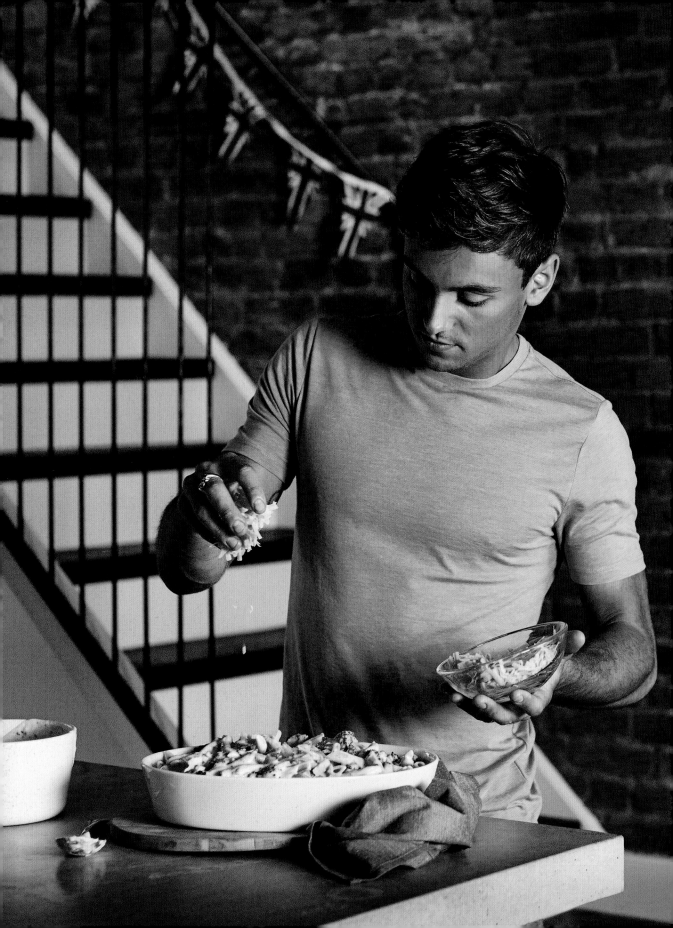

WEEKEND FEASTS

~ STUFFED SUMMER VEG ~

I love that this recipe combines animal and vegetable protein – the lentils add good fibre and make the meat stretch a little further. If you don't eat all the vegetables for supper they are good cold the next day so just right for lunch with a salad.

SERVES 2

438 CALORIES PER SERVING

1 tbsp olive oil

1 shallot, chopped

1 aubergine, halved through the core

1 large courgette, halved through the core

1 garlic clove, chopped

1 tsp cumin seeds, roughly crushed

½ cinnamon stick or ¼–½ tsp ground cinnamon

1 tbsp freshly chopped thyme or ½ tsp dried thyme

125g lean pork mince

50g red lentils

2 large plum tomatoes (about 200g), chopped, or use 200g chopped tomatoes from a can

350ml hot chicken or vegetable stock

3 dried apricots (about 30g), chopped (optional)

1 pepper (red, green or yellow), halved and deseeded

15g whole almonds, chopped

2 tbsp freshly chopped parsley

salt and freshly ground black pepper

1 Preheat the oven to 200°C/180°C Fan/Gas 6. Heat the oil in a pan and cook the shallot over a low to medium heat for 5 minutes.

2 Scoop the seeds and middle out of the aubergine, leaving a channel in the middle and about 1cm of flesh round the outside. Then take the courgette halves and use a teaspoon to scrape out the seeds from the middle. Chop all the bits of vegetable you've scooped out and put them in the pan with the shallot. Stir in the garlic, spices and thyme and cook for 2–3 minutes.

3 Add the pork mince to the pan with the red lentils and the chopped tomatoes. Cook for a few minutes, then add the hot stock and the chopped apricots, if using. Cover the pan and cook for 5 minutes, then take the lid off and continue to simmer for 15 minutes. Put the aubergine, courgette and pepper halves in an ovenproof dish and pop them into the oven for 15 minutes.

4 Take the vegetables out of the oven and divide the pork and lentil sauce evenly between them. If you've used a cinnamon stick, remove and discard it.

5 Sprinkle the chopped almonds over the stuffed vegetables, season them well, then put them in the oven for 30 minutes until tender. Sprinkle with the parsley and serve with a green salad.

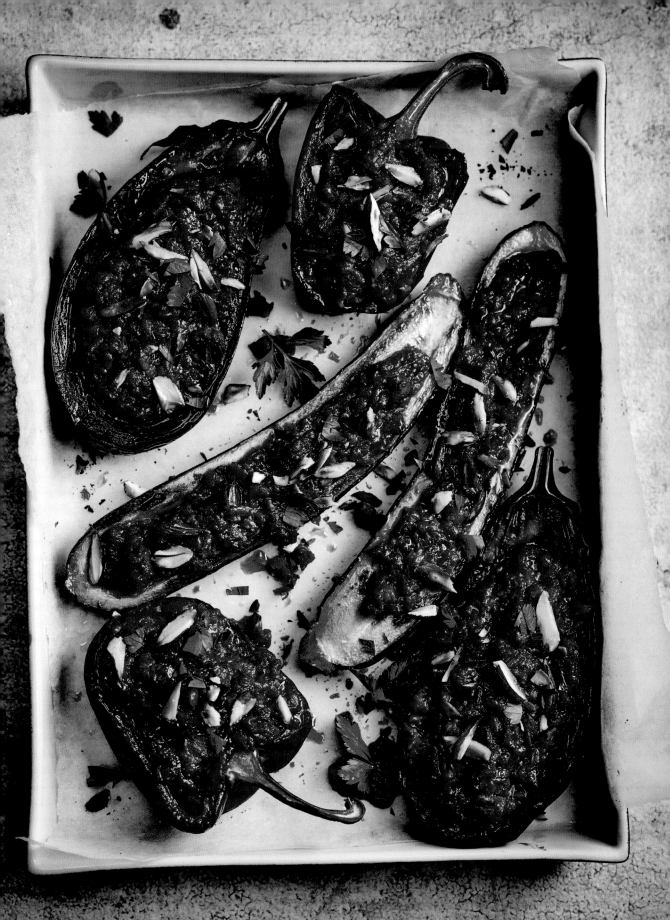

≈ VEGGIE BURGERS ≈

These spicy veggie burgers are served on guilt-free baked mushrooms instead
of buns, but you still get that great burger feeling – especially if you treat yourself
to some mayo and ketchup! Serve with crunchy sweet potato chips for a real feast.

SERVES 2

416 CALORIES PER SERVING

2 tsp olive oil, plus extra
for brushing

1 shallot, finely chopped

1 carrot, diced

1 celery stick, diced

125g butternut squash, diced

1 tsp ground coriander

½ tsp dried oregano

¼–½ tsp cayenne pepper
(depending on how hot you like
your food)

400g can of white beans,
drained well

3 small slices of wholemeal
bread (about 65g), whizzed
into crumbs

4 large Portobello mushrooms

1 large sweet potato
(250g), unpeeled

8–10 cherry tomatoes, halved
and a few basil leaves, to serve

ketchup and mayonnaise
(optional), to serve

salt and freshly ground
black pepper

1 Heat the oil in a saucepan and add the
shallot, carrot, celery and squash with
3 tablespoons of water. Season well, cover
the pan and gently cook the vegetables for
15 minutes, stirring occasionally, until they're
very soft. Stir in the spices and beans, then
cook for 1 minute. Remove the pan from
the heat and leave to cool.

2 Tip half the mixture into a food processor
and whizz until it forms a rough purée.
Tip this purée into a bowl, add the remaining
mixture and half the breadcrumbs. Season
again and stir everything together. Spoon
the remaining breadcrumbs into a bowl.

3 Divide the mixture roughly into 4. Shape
a portion into a burger, then toss it in the
bowl of breadcrumbs to coat. Repeat to
shape and coat the rest of the burgers.

4 Preheat oven to 200°C/180°C Fan/Gas 6.
Cut the sweet potato into thin chips,
about 9cm x 1cm in size. Put the chips on
a roasting tray, brush them with oil, season
them well and roast for 10 minutes. Then
add the burgers to the tray – handle them
carefully as they will be quite soft – and
continue to roast for another 20 minutes.

5 Ten minutes before the end of the
cooking time, put the mushrooms
on a baking tray, brush them with oil
and season them with salt and pepper.
Put them in the oven with the burgers
and sweet potato chips.

6 Serve each burger on a mushroom with
the sweet potato chips, cherry tomatoes
and basil leaves and a dollop of ketchup
and/or mayo if you like.

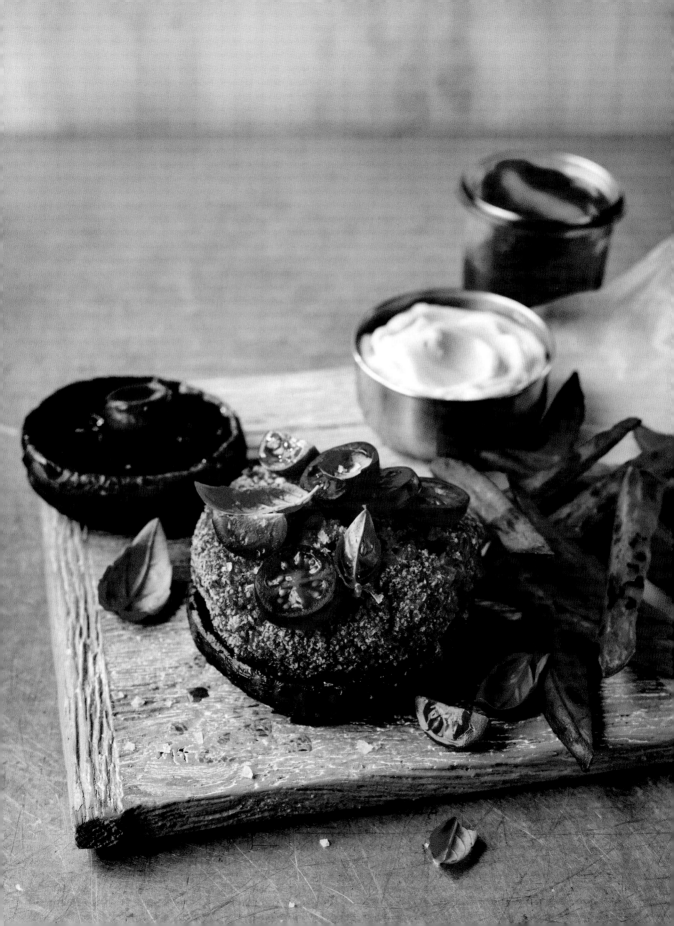

≈ HEALTHY CRÊPES ≈
WITH THREE QUICK FILLINGS

I'm a big fan of crêpes and these are very thin and light. I love experimenting with different healthy and nutritious fillings so here are some of my favourites!

SERVES 2

20g each of plain flour and wholemeal flour

1 medium egg

150ml milk

drizzle of olive oil

NO-COOK FILLING

311 CALORIES PER SERVING

300g cooked shelled prawns

4 tbsp natural yoghurt

100g cucumber, finely sliced

salt and black pepper

5-MINUTE FILLING

346 CALORIES PER SERVING

2 tsp olive oil

100g mushrooms, finely sliced

100g spinach, chopped

50g mature Cheddar, grated

2 tbsp natural yoghurt

10-MINUTE FILLING

487 CALORIES PER SERVING

1 tsp oil

1 shallot, chopped

½ pepper, deseeded and chopped

2 skinless salmon fillets (about 125g each), chopped

1 tbsp capers

2 tbsp natural yoghurt

small handful of freshly chopped chives

1 Put the plain and wholemeal flour into a bowl and stir. Add the egg and milk and mix everything together, taking care not to overbeat the mixture. Set the batter aside for 30 minutes, then give it a good stir again.

2 Heat a 20cm frying pan over a medium heat. Add a drop of olive oil and wipe it round the pan with kitchen paper. Add 4 tablespoons of batter, swirl it around, then cook the crêpe for about 2 minutes. Slide it on to a plate and repeat to make 3 more.

3 For the no-cook filling, just mix all the ingredients and season well. Divide the filling between the crêpes and fold them up.

4 For the 5-minute filling, heat the oil in a pan and cook the mushrooms for a few minutes until golden. Add the spinach, allow it to wilt, then stir in the cheese and yoghurt and season well. Divide the filling between the crêpes and fold them up.

5 For the 10-minute filling, heat the oil in a pan and stir-fry the shallot and pepper for 2–3 minutes. Season well, then stir in the salmon and capers and cook for a further 3–4 minutes until everything is just cooked through. Divide the filling between the crêpes, top each crêpe with half a tablespoon of yoghurt and scatter over the chives. Fold up the crêpes.

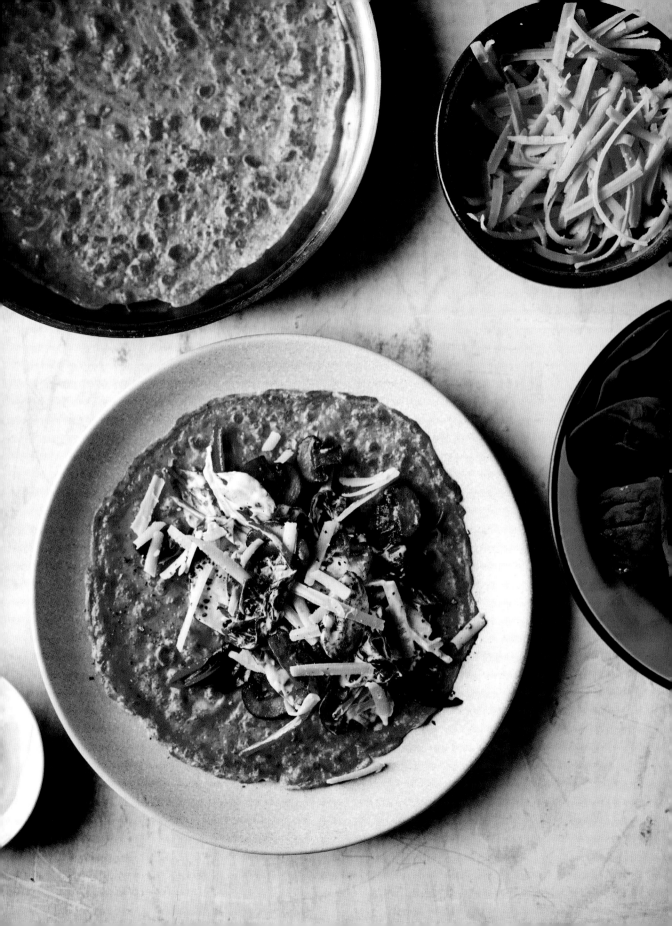

≈ NAN'S BROCCOLI BAKE ≈

This is my Nan's special recipe and she always used to cook it for us when we were little. Everyone loves it and it's packed with good stuff. Nan always makes sure she seasons the sauce well and she uses strong Cheddar for the best flavour.

SERVES 6

447 CALORIES PER SERVING

40g butter

40g plain flour

400ml each of milk and hot vegetable stock, measured together in a jug

150g mature Cheddar cheese, grated

small handful of parsley, finely chopped

grating of nutmeg

300g penne pasta

300g broccoli, chopped, including the stalk

1 carrot, diced

100g frozen peas

salt and freshly ground black pepper

1 Bring a large saucepan of salted water to the boil. While you're waiting for the water to boil, make the cheese sauce. Melt the butter in a medium saucepan and stir in the flour. Cook for 1–2 minutes until the mixture forms a paste and starts to bubble on the bottom of the pan. Whip the pan off the heat and slowly add the milk and stock mixture, stirring all the time until you have a smooth sauce.

2 Place the pan back over the heat, keeping it very low, and stir constantly until the sauce thickens and coats the back of the spoon. Stir in three quarters of the cheese, add the parsley and season with nutmeg and salt and pepper. Preheat the oven to 200°C/180°C Fan/Gas 6.

3 Add the pasta to the pan of boiling water and cook it according to the packet instructions. About 5 minutes before the end of the cooking time, add the broccoli and carrot. Cover and bring the water back to the boil quickly, then remove the lid again and cook for the remaining time. Drop the peas into the pan – they'll thaw immediately in the boiling water. Drain everything well and tip the whole lot back into the pan.

4 Pour the cheese sauce on top of the pasta mixture and give everything a good stir so it's all well coated. Transfer the mixture to a large ovenproof dish (about 3 litres). Scatter the remaining cheese evenly over the top and bake for 25–30 minutes or until the top is brown and crispy.

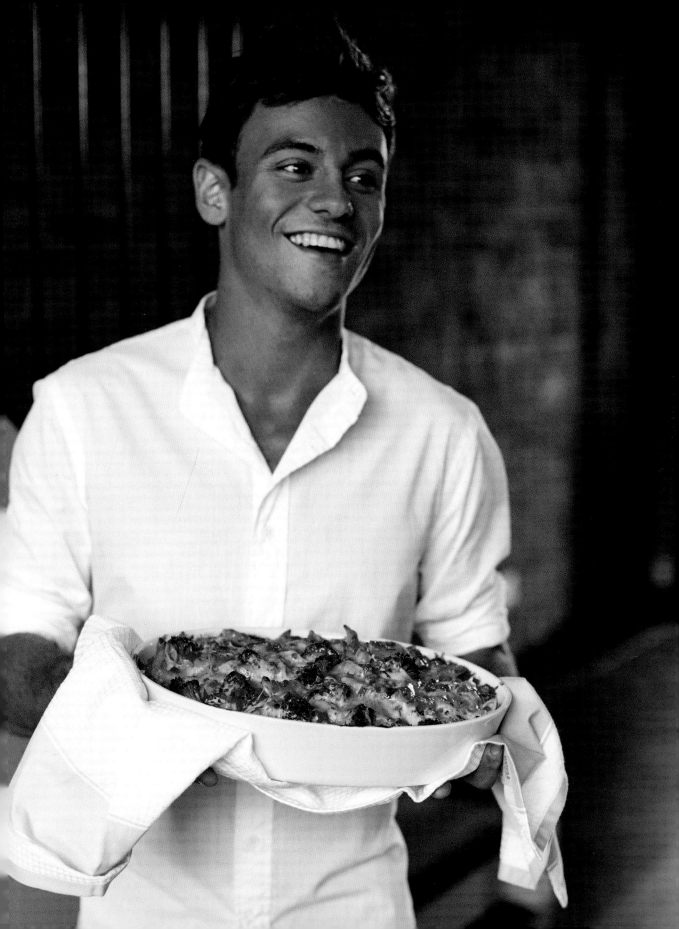

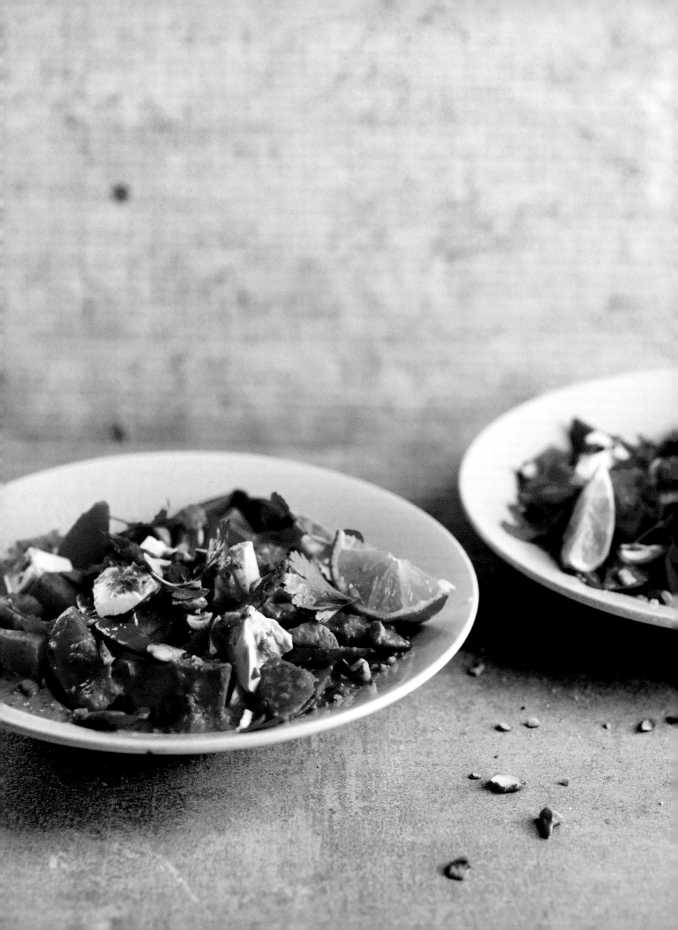

～ THAI-STYLE CURRY ～
WITH TOFU

There are Thai curry pastes in every supermarket, but I've discovered that it's really simple to make your own – and if I can do it so can you! Home-made paste has loads more flavour and is much healthier than the shop-bought versions. I wasn't sure about tofu at first but it's great in this curry and it's very easy to use. If you're not a tofu fan, you could add leftover cooked chicken or prawns or even some thinly sliced roast beef instead.

SERVES 2

290 CALORIES PER SERVING

1 sweet potato, diced

65g coconut cream

250ml hot vegetable or chicken stock

100g mangetout, halved

1 pak choi, sliced lengthways

½ red pepper, deseeded and sliced

175g silken tofu (about ½ pack, roughly broken up

½ lime, cut into 2 wedges

CURRY PASTE

1 shallot, chopped

zest and juice of 1 lime

10g fresh root ginger, peeled

10g fresh coriander, roughly chopped, plus a few extra leaves to garnish

1 tbsp coconut oil

1 red chilli, halved and deseeded – if you like a hot paste, add the seeds

½ tsp salt

1 Put all the ingredients for the curry paste into a small food processor and whizz until smooth.

2 Put 2 tablespoons of the paste into a wok and cook over a medium heat for about 1 minute. Add the sweet potato and toss it in the mixture, then cook for 1 minute.

3 Add the coconut cream and stock and bring to a simmer. Cook over a low heat for 5–10 minutes until the sweet potato is just tender.

4 Add the remaining vegetables, cover the wok with a lid and cook for about 5 minutes until all the vegetables are tender. Taste to check the seasoning. If the sauce is very thick, stir in 50–100ml of hot water.

5 Divide the curry between 2 bowls, top with the silken tofu and a few coriander leaves and serve with the lime wedges.

≈
TOM'S TIP

The recipe makes more curry paste than you need for this dish, but it can be stored in a jar in the fridge for up to 2 weeks.

≈

≈ TOM'S FABULOUS FAJITAS ≈

My famous fajitas always go down brilliantly when my friends come over. I love adding lots of different salad bits to sprinkle over the top, like beans, peppers, sweetcorn and guacamole. You can double or treble this recipe if you want.

SERVES 2

669 CALORIES PER SERVING

MARINATED CHICKEN

½ tsp cayenne

½ tsp dried oregano

½ tsp paprika

½ tsp ground coriander

¼ tsp ground cinnamon

grating of nutmeg

250g skinless, boneless chicken (thighs or breasts), sliced into thin strips

1 small red onion, sliced

1 garlic clove, sliced

1 tbsp olive oil

salt and freshly ground black pepper

BEAN, SWEETCORN AND PEPPER SALAD

1 corn on the cob, husk removed

½ red pepper, diced

½ can of beans (use black, kidney or cannellini), drained

½ quantity of salsa (see p.29)

GUACAMOLE

½ avocado, flesh chopped

zest and juice of ½ lime

½ red chilli, chopped

TO SERVE

4 wholemeal tortilla wraps

½ cos lettuce, cut into wedges

small handful of chopped fresh coriander

extra chilli, finely sliced (optional)

2 tbsp soured cream (optional)

1 Start by marinating the chicken – you can do this up to 8 hours ahead. Put the cayenne, oregano, paprika, coriander, cinnamon and nutmeg in a bowl. Add the chicken, onion, garlic and a teaspoon of olive oil, then season well and toss everything together.

2 Bring a medium pan of water to the boil and cook the corn on the cob for about 3 minutes until the corn is cooked. Add the pepper to the pan to blanch it, then drain well. Leave the corn cob until it's cool enough to handle, then carefully slice the kernels from the cob. Put the corn, pepper and beans into a bowl, add the salsa and season the salad well.

3 To make the guacamole, mash the avocado in a bowl until smooth. Stir in the lime zest, juice and the chilli and season. Set it aside.

4 Cook the chicken. Heat the remaining oil in a pan and stir-fry the chicken for 13–15 minutes until golden and cooked through.

5 Put 2 wraps on each plate, then spoon on the chicken, bean salad, guacamole, lettuce, coriander, chilli and soured cream. Roll the wraps up and enjoy.

TOM'S TIP
If you want to use a ready-made fajita spice blend, use 1–2 teaspoons instead of the spices listed above.

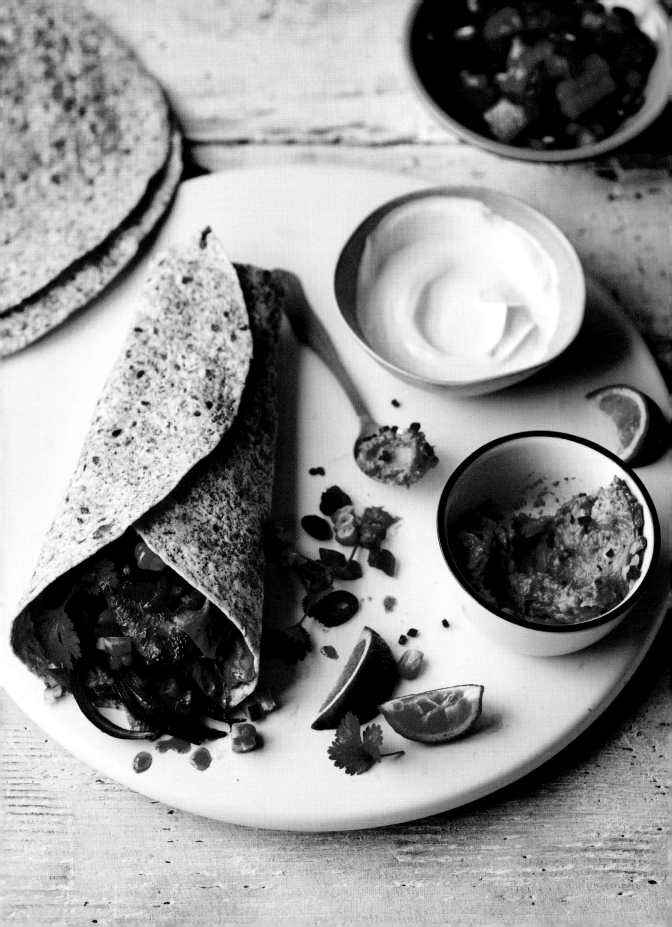

≈ CHICKEN AND BACON PARCELS ≈

This recipe turns a couple of ordinary chicken breasts into a real treat. It looks impressive but it's not difficult to prepare. Pancetta is just Italian-style bacon and if you can't find any, you can use streaky bacon rashers instead. And if you have some canned beans left over from the Fajita-stuffed chicken (see page 96), this is a great way to use them up!

SERVES 2

407 CALORIES PER SERVING

2 spring onions, finely chopped

2 tbsp full-fat cream cheese

2 small skinless chicken breasts

a few sprigs of thyme

60g pancetta (6–8 rashers)

160g mixed beans from a can, drained and rinsed

2 tomatoes, chopped

small handful of basil, freshly chopped, plus extra to garnish

salt and freshly ground black pepper

1 Put the spring onions and cream cheese in a bowl, season them with salt and pepper and mix well.

2 Place a chicken breast on a board with the smooth side down. Slice through it horizontally, but don't cut right through to the other side, then open it out like a book. Repeat with the other breast.

3 Season the chicken breasts well, then divide the cream cheese mixture between them. Roll up each chicken breast, season them and put a little thyme on each one.

4 Take 3 or 4 pieces of pancetta and wrap them around one of the rolled-up chicken breasts so the meat is completely covered. Do the same with the other piece of chicken and the remaining pancetta.

5 Heat a frying pan until hot and add the parcels. Brown them all over for about 8 minutes in total until golden. Add a couple of tablespoons of boiling water and cover the pan with a lid. Cook for 15–20 minutes over a low heat until the chicken is cooked through and no pink juices remain. Lift the parcels out of the pan and set them aside on a plate.

6 Put the mixed beans and tomatoes into the pan with the basil. Stir everything into the juices in the pan and warm through. Season well.

7 Divide the bean mixture between 2 plates and top with the chicken. Drizzle over any juices from the rested chicken and garnish with extra basil, then serve at once.

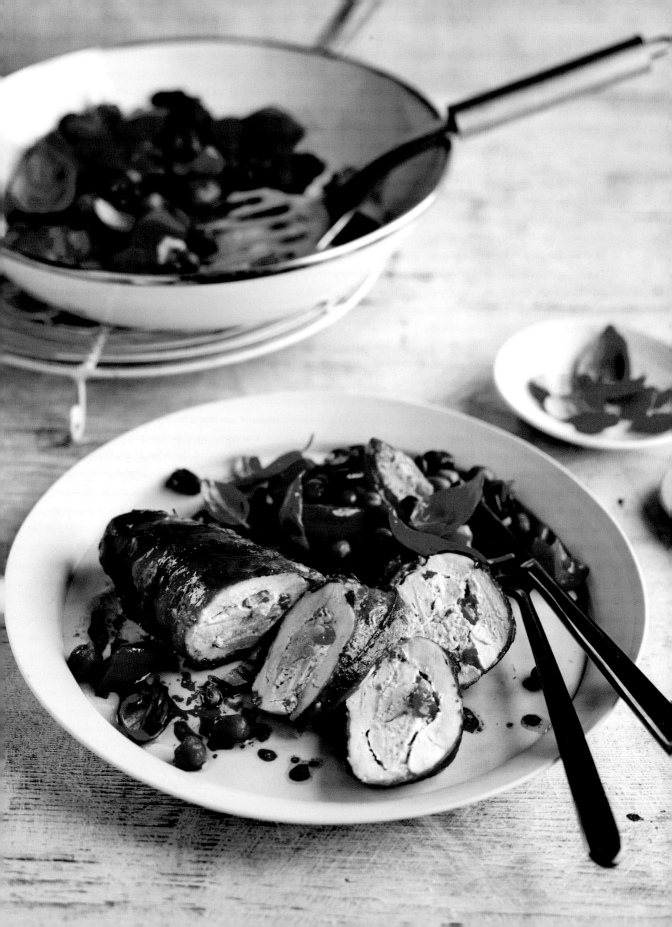

≈ TOM'S BIG BARBECUE TREAT ≈

Lance and I love barbecuing – Lance barbecues even when it's freezing outside and he has to wear his hat and gloves! Here is a selection of our favourite BBQ treats – make the whole lot for a real feast. I hope you enjoy them as much as we do.

SWEET CHILLI PRAWNS OR PORK

SERVES 6

82 CALORIES PER SERVING WITH PRAWNS

106 CALORIES PER SERVING WITH PORK

¼–½ tsp chilli flakes

1 fat garlic clove, crushed

1 tbsp honey

2 tsp tomato purée

2 tbsp olive oil

1 tsp rice wine vinegar or white wine vinegar

300g raw shelled prawns or 300g chopped pork fillet

salt and freshly ground black pepper

1 Mix the chilli flakes, garlic, honey, tomato purée, oil and vinegar together in a bowl and season well. Add the prawns or pork and set aside for 30 minutes.

2 To cook the prawns, thread them on to 6 skewers and grill them on the barbecue until they change from grey to pink, turning them once. They'll take 3–4 minutes.

3 For the pork, thread the pieces on to 6 skewers. Cook the pork on the barbecue for about 15 minutes until cooked through, turning the skewers half way through the cooking time.

SOY AND GINGER CHICKEN

SERVES 6

84 CALORIES PER SERVING

1 tbsp coconut oil

2 tsp sesame oil

2 tsp soy sauce

15g fresh root ginger, grated

zest and juice of 1 lime

1 tsp honey

300g chicken mini fillets

salt and freshly ground black pepper

1 Mix the oils, soy sauce, ginger, lime zest and juice and the honey together in a bowl and season well. Add the chicken mini fillets and set aside for 30 minutes.

2 Divide the chicken pieces between 6 skewers. Cook them on the barbecue for about 10 minutes, turning once. To check the chicken is properly cooked, slice through the thickest piece – it should be white inside with no pink juices.

≈
TOM'S TIP
If you use wooden skewers, soak them in water for at least half an hour first so they don't burn on the barbecue.
≈

SAUSAGES WITH HONEY AND LEMON DRESSING

SERVES 6

236 CALORIES PER SERVING

1 tbsp honey

zest and juice of 1 lemon

2 tbsp olive oil

small handful of freshly chopped parsley

6 good-quality pork sausages

salt and freshly ground black pepper

1 Put the honey, lemon zest and juice, olive oil and parsley into a bowl and season well. Set aside while you barbecue the sausages.

2 As soon as the sausages are ready – they'll take 20–30 minutes to cook – put them on a plate and spoon the honey and lemon dressing over the top.

CRISPY ASPARAGUS

SERVES 6

29 CALORIES PER SERVING

250g asparagus spears (thin ones work best)

1 tbsp coconut oil

salt and freshly ground black pepper

1 Brush the asparagus with coconut oil or if you find it easier, massage the oil into the spears.

2 Put the asparagus spears on the barbecue and grill them until they're golden and cooked through, then season and serve.

THE PERFECT CHOPPED SALAD

SERVES 6

41 CALORIES PER SERVING

2 celery sticks, finely sliced

1 little gem lettuce or ½ cos, finely sliced

½ fennel bulb, finely chopped

75g cucumber, chopped

75g white cabbage, finely chopped

3 tbsp freshly chopped parsley

DRESSING

2 tbsp extra virgin olive oil

2 tbsp mayonnaise

1½ tbsp red or white wine vinegar

salt and freshly ground black pepper

1 Put all the ingredients for the dressing into a large bowl and season well. Mix everything together.

2 Add the celery, lettuce, fennel, cucumber, cabbage and parsley to the bowl and stir everything together.

SIMPLE BEAN SALAD

SERVES 6

138 CALORIES PER SERVING

2 x 400g cans of mixed beans, drained well

200g cherry tomatoes, halved

large handful of freshly chopped parsley

1 chilli, halved, deseeded and very finely chopped

2 tbsp extra virgin olive oil

½ tbsp red wine vinegar

salt and freshly ground black pepper

Put all the ingredients into a large bowl, season with salt and pepper, then mix well.

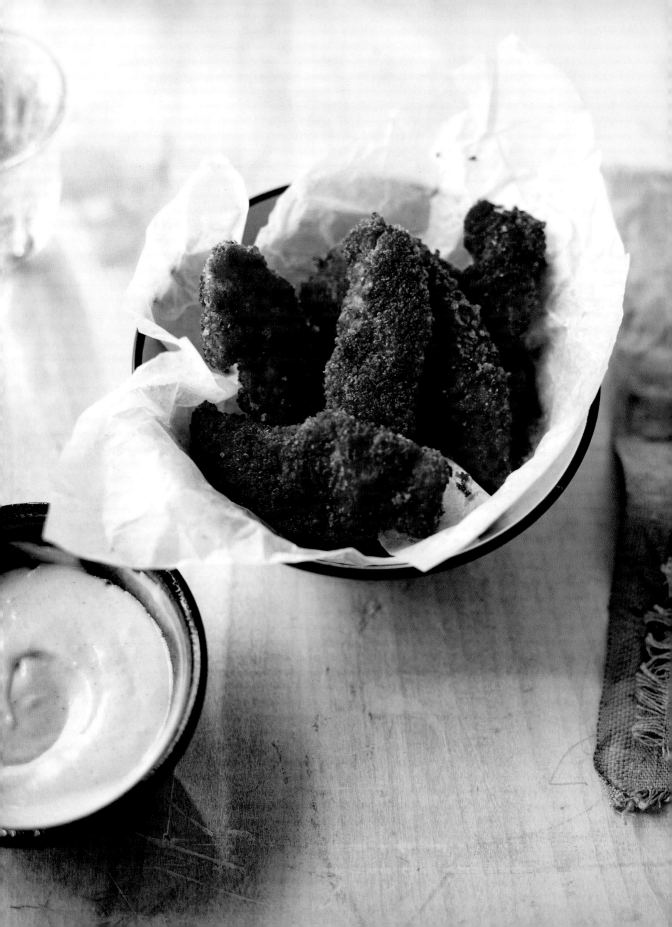

~ SOUTHERN FRIED CHICKEN ~
WITH WHITE GRAVY

This is what Lance always makes for me as a treat when I've finished a competition.
It's a favourite dish in the southern US and everyone has their own take on how
to make white gravy – which is similar to a white sauce. I've taken this classic
and given it some healthy adjustments for a scrumptious dinner!

SERVES 2

551 CALORIES PER SERVING

1 tbsp plain flour

1 medium egg, beaten

75g wholemeal breadcrumbs

250g chicken mini fillets

2 tbsp olive oil

WHITE GRAVY

15g butter

15g flour

250ml milk

salt, freshly ground black pepper and white pepper

1 Put the flour, egg and breadcrumbs into separate bowls and season each with salt and pepper. Take a strip of chicken and toss it first in the flour, then in the beaten egg and lastly in the breadcrumbs. Do the same with the rest of the pieces. Preheat the oven to 180°C/160°C Fan/Gas 4.

2 Heat a tablespoon of the oil in a pan and fry a few of the chicken pieces on each side until golden – it's important not to overcrowd the pan or the chicken will steam and not fry properly. Transfer the chicken to a baking tray and continue to fry the rest, in batches, transferring each batch to the tray once it is browned. Put the chicken in the oven for 10 minutes to cook it through.

3 Make the white gravy. Melt the butter in a small pan and stir in the flour. Cook for 1–2 minutes, making sure the flour doesn't turn brown.

4 Slowly add the milk and stir well until smooth. Season well with salt and white pepper, then simmer the sauce for 2–3 minutes until it has thickened slightly.

5 Serve the chicken with the white gravy and some green vegetables.

≈ MUM'S SUNDAY LUNCH ≈

When I think of Sundays, I think of roast dinners. Sunday has always been my day off and when I lived at home, we always had the family round for a roast. Now I cook my own and I find that the trickiest thing is getting everything ready at the same time, so I follow my mum's method. It always works. Of course, you don't have to cook all the dishes but if you do, you'll have a treat – and probably some leftovers for Monday!

SERVES 6

753 CALORIES PER SERVING

1 chicken (about 1.8 kg)

½ lemon

sprig each of rosemary, sage and thyme

2 tbsp olive oil

200ml reserved potato water

20g plain flour

800ml–1 litre reserved vegetable water

salt and freshly ground black pepper

ROAST POTATOES

700g fluffy potatoes, such as King Edwards or Maris Pipers

1 onion, halved and each cut into three wedges

3 tbsp olive oil

BROCCOLI, LEEK AND COURGETTE CHEESE BAKE

250g broccoli, chopped

300g leek (1 large), chopped

300g courgette (about 2), chopped

20g butter

20g plain flour

200ml milk

200ml reserved vegetable water

110g mature Cheddar cheese, grated

MASHED POTATO AND SWEDE

350g swede, chopped

300g sweet potato, chopped

20g butter

CARROTS AND PEAS

200g carrots, sliced

200g frozen peas

10g butter

small handful of freshly chopped parsley

TOM'S TIP

Mum always uses the veg cooking water in her gravy and cheese sauce. The water is full of nutrients and the starch in it helps to thicken the sauces, so it's a shame to chuck it down the sink.

≈

1 Preheat the oven to 200°C/180°C Fan/ Gas 6. Put the chicken in a roasting tin and push the lemon and herbs into the cavity. Pour 300ml of cold water into the tin and drizzle the oil over the chicken. Season well. Calculate the cooking time – the chicken will need 20 minutes for every 450g, plus an extra 20 minutes, so for a 1.8kg bird, that's 1 hour and 40 minutes. After 1 hour, add the 200ml of reserved potato water (see below) to the pan.

2 Once the chicken is in the oven, put the potatoes into a saucepan and pour in enough cold water to cover them. Put a lid on the pan and bring it to the boil. When the water is boiling, turn the heat down slightly and cook the potatoes for about 6 minutes. Add the wedges of onion to the pan to blanch them, then drain everything well, reserving the water. Shake the potatoes in a colander to roughen up the edges. Heat the oil in a roasting tin and add the potatoes (save the onions to add later). Season the potatoes well and toss to coat them in the oil. Put them in the oven to roast for 1 hour.

3 Bring a large pan of water to the boil. Once it's boiling, add the broccoli and leek and cook for 3 minutes, then add the courgette and cook for 1 minute. Drain, reserving the vegetable water. Arrange the vegetables in an ovenproof dish.

4 Make the cheese sauce. Melt the butter in a pan and add the flour, then stir over a low heat for 1 minute. Slowly add the milk and veg water, stirring all the time until smooth. Stir in half the cheese and season. Spoon the sauce over the vegetables and scatter the remaining cheese on top. Cook in the oven for 30 minutes until golden.

5 For the mash, put the swede in a pan and cover it with cold water. Cook it for 15 minutes, then add the sweet potato and cook for 10 minutes more until everything is tender. Drain well, again reserving the vegetable water. Return the veg to the pan, add the butter, then season and mash well. Cover the pan and keep the mash warm.

6 Check the chicken is cooked by pushing a skewer into the thigh. If the juices are clear, it's ready. If not, put the chicken back in the oven and check every 5 minutes. Once the chicken is done, put it on a warm plate, making sure that all the juices are poured into the roasting tin. Cover the chicken with foil and set it aside to rest.

7 Add the onions to the roast potatoes and continue to roast them for about 15 minutes while you make the gravy.

8 To make the gravy, drain off all but about a tablespoon of fat from the roasting tin, leaving the juices in the tin. Add the flour and cook over a low heat for 1–2 minutes. Slowly add 800ml–1 litre of vegetable water and stir well to make a smooth sauce. Slowly bring the gravy to a simmer and cook for 10–15 minutes until it is syrupy.

9 Cook the carrots in a pan of boiling water until they're just tender. Add the peas and cook for 1–2 minutes more. Drain the vegetables well, return them to the pan and add the butter, parsley and seasoning. Cover and keep warm.

10 Carve the chicken and serve with all the vegetables and the gravy.

≈ CHICKEN SKEWERS ≈
WITH ROASTED VEGETABLES

Chicken skewers are great party food: they're fun and easy to eat with your hands – and they're really healthy too. You can marinate the chicken up to a day ahead if you like. Store it in the fridge and take it out 30 minutes before you want to cook it.

SERVES 2

603 CALORIES PER SERVING

2 tsp smoked paprika

2 tsp dried oregano or marjoram

1 tsp hot paprika

good pinch of chilli flakes

zest and juice of 1 lemon

2 tbsp olive oil

2 chicken breasts (about 300g), chopped into chunks

1 sweet potato (about 150g), chopped into large chunks

1 courgette (about 120g), sliced into chunks

¼ cauliflower or broccoli (about 120g), sliced in half

1 red onion (about 100g), quartered

½ red pepper, deseeded and cut into 4 pieces

salt and freshly ground black pepper

QUINOA

100g quinoa

300ml hot vegetable stock

small handful of freshly chopped herbs, such as parsley, coriander, chives and mint

TO SERVE

10g flaked almonds, toasted

2 tbsp natural yoghurt

1 Preheat the oven to 190°C/170°C Fan/Gas 5. Put a teaspoon of paprika, a teaspoon of dried oregano or marjoram, half a teaspoon of hot paprika, some chilli flakes, the lemon zest and juice and a tablespoon of olive oil in a bowl. Season well and stir everything together. Add the chicken and set it aside to marinate.

2 In a separate bowl, stir together the remaining spices and herbs. Stir in a tablespoon of oil and 3 tablespoons of water, then add the prepared vegetables and season them well. Toss everything to coat it all in the spice mixture, then tip it into a roasting tin and roast for 35–40 minutes.

3 After 15 minutes, remove the chicken from the marinade and push the pieces on to metal skewers. Put them on a baking tray, drizzle over any remaining marinade and cook in the oven on the shelf under the vegetables for 20 minutes.

4 Put the quinoa in an ovenproof pan and pour in the stock. Cover the pan and bring the stock to the boil on the hob. Put the pan in the oven for 20 minutes until the quinoa has absorbed all the liquid.

5 Fluff up the quinoa and stir in the herbs. Serve it with the roasted veg and the chicken and garnish with flaked almonds. Serve the yoghurt on the side.

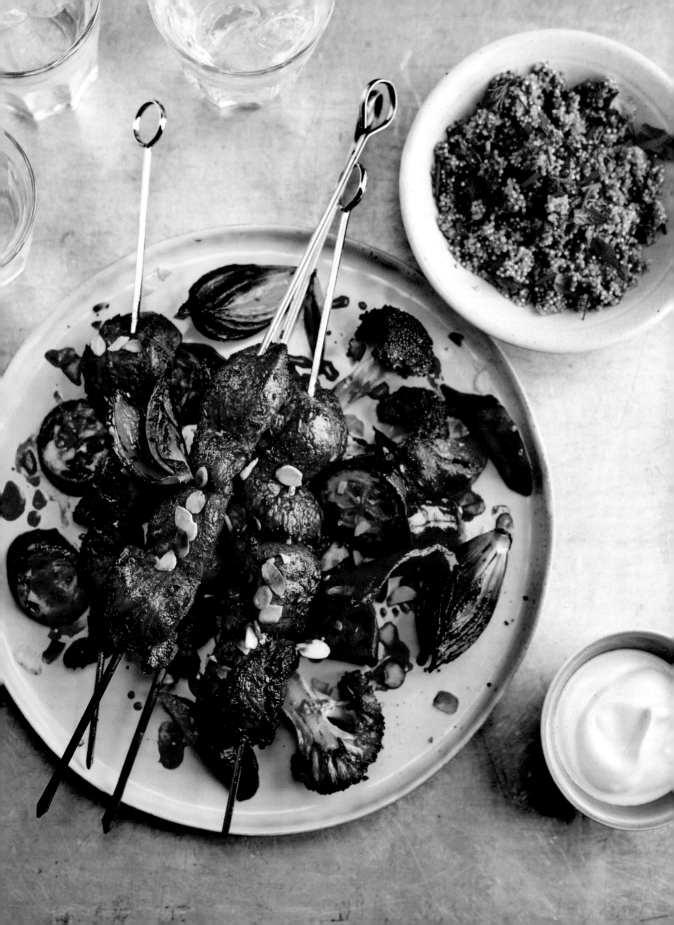

≈ TURKEY MEATBALLS ≈
WITH COURGETTI

I like turkey and find it a good healthy alternative to beef, as it's lower in fat, calories and cholesterol. The couscous makes these meatballs really filling and adds extra texture. Spiralised courgettes (courgetti) make an ideal side dish or you could serve them with a tomato salsa or just a salad.

SERVES 2

300 CALORIES PER SERVING

25g wholemeal couscous

1 shallot, chopped

250g turkey breast meat

1 tbsp freshly chopped sage

1 medium egg

zest of ½ lemon

good pinch of chilli flakes

1½ tsp olive oil

250ml hot vegetable or chicken stock

2 medium courgettes (about 300g)

5g butter

salt and freshly ground black pepper

1 Put the couscous in a large bowl, add 25ml of just-boiled water and leave it to soak. Fluff the couscous up with a fork.

2 Put the shallot, turkey, sage, egg, lemon zest and chilli into a food processor and season well. Whizz until all the ingredients are chopped and the mixture looks minced.

3 Tip everything into the bowl with the couscous and mix all the ingredients together. Divide the mixture into 6 portions and shape each into a ball.

4 Heat the oil in a large frying pan and brown the balls until they're golden all over. You may need to do this in batches, setting each batch aside while you brown the next. Put all the meatballs back in the pan and add the stock, then cover the pan with a lid and simmer for about 15 minutes, turning the balls half way through.

5 Cut the courgettes into ribbons using a Y peeler or a spiraliser. Put the courgetti into a pan with a little water. Bring to the boil and steam until the courgetti are tender. Drain them well, add the butter and season, then serve with the turkey boulders.

TOM'S TIP
This mixture can also be made into mini meatballs. Follow the recipe and shape the mixture into 16 pieces – each a little bigger than a golf ball. To cook, fry the meatballs in batches until golden, then simmer in the stock for about 10 minutes. Cut a meatball in half to check it's cooked through before serving.
≈

≈ SPICY COTTAGE PIE ≈
WITH A MEXICAN TWIST

My special twist on the classic cottage pie has a spicy Mexican vibe and it's so delicious, you'll never look back! All you need is a crisp salad on the side. For an extra Mexican touch, squeeze some fresh lime juice over your pie when you serve it. Awesome.

SERVES 2

518 CALORIES PER SERVING

1 tbsp olive oil

1 small red onion, chopped

1 carrot, chopped

1 celery stick, chopped

½ red pepper, chopped

1 garlic clove, chopped

200g lean mince

½ tsp dried chilli flakes

1 tsp dried or 2 tsp fresh oregano

1 tsp paprika

1 tsp ground cumin

200g chopped tomatoes

200ml hot vegetable, chicken or beef stock

½ tbsp tomato purée

½ can black beans (about 100g) drained

300g sweet potato, chopped

10g butter

15g mature Cheddar cheese, grated

salt and freshly ground black pepper

1 Heat a teaspoon of the oil in a pan and add the onion, carrot, celery and pepper, then a tablespoon of water. Season well. Cover the pan and cook over a low to medium heat for 10 minutes. Stir every now and then to stop the vegetables from burning. Stir in the garlic and cook for 1 minute, then spoon the mixture on to a plate.

2 Add the remaining oil to the pan and add about a third of the mince. Place the pan over a medium heat and brown the mince by pushing it down with the back of a wooden spoon to cover the base of the pan. Allow it to cook for a couple of minutes until it's golden, then turn it over and do the other side. Break it up with the tip of the spoon until it looks crumbly. Spoon the mince on to the plate with the veg, then cook the rest in the same way in a couple of batches.

3 Put the vegetables and meat back in the pan and add the chilli and spices. Season well and cook for a couple of minutes. Stir in the tomatoes, stock, pureé and beans, cover the pan and bring to a simmer. Cook for about 45 minutes until the mince is tender.

4 After about 25 minutes, preheat the oven to 200°C/180°C Fan/Gas 6. Put the sweet potato in a pan of cold water, then bring to the boil. Turn the heat down to a simmer and cook the sweet potato for 10–15 minutes until tender. Drain, then tip it back into the pan, season and mash with the butter.

5 Spoon the mince and vegetables into an 800ml–1 litre ovenproof dish and cover with the mash. Scatter the cheese on top and bake the pie in the oven for about 20 minutes until golden on top and piping hot.

≈ MUM'S SAUSAGE CASSEROLE ≈

Lots of people assume sausages are unhealthy, but as long as you choose
good-quality ones with a high meat content, they're fine once in a while. This
recipe was a firm favourite with my brothers and me when we were growing up
and I often cook it for myself now. I like to serve it with root vegetable mash.

SERVES 2

500 CALORIES PER SERVING

1 tsp olive oil

1 red onion, cut into thick
wedges

3–4 sprigs of thyme

1 garlic clove, sliced

4 pork and herb sausages

5g butter

15g plain flour

250ml hot beef stock

1 tsp tomato purée

good splash of Worcestershire
sauce

small handful of freshly
chopped parsley, to serve

salt and freshly ground black
pepper

ROOT VEGETABLE MASH

1 parsnip (about 125g), chopped

1 large carrot (about 125g),
chopped

150g wedge of swede, chopped

50ml milk

10g butter

1 Heat the oil in a flameproof casserole dish
and stir-fry the red onion for 5 minutes
until it starts to soften. Stir in the thyme and
garlic, season well, and cook for 1 minute.

2 Add the sausages to the pan and brown
them on each side. Take the onion and
sausages out of the pan and set them aside.
Add the butter and plain flour and stir for
about a minute to make a paste. Slowly add
the stock, stirring constantly to make a
smooth sauce. Stir in the tomato purée
and Worcestershire sauce.

3 Put the onions and sausages back in the
pan and put the lid on. Bring to a gentle
simmer, then cook for 20–25 minutes,
stirring every now and then.

4 To make the mash, put the root veg in
a saucepan, cover them with cold water
and add salt. Put a lid on the pan and bring
to the boil. Simmer for about 20–25 minutes
until all the vegetables are very tender. Drain
them, then tip them back into the pan. Put
the pan back on the turned-off hob and leave
for a minute or so to steam-dry the veg. Add
the milk and butter, then season and mash
until smooth.

5 Serve the mash with the sausages and
spoon the gravy over the top. Garnish
with parsley and serve with green veg.

TOM'S TIP
Mum used to serve this with potato
mash. Use 400g of floury potatoes,
such as King Edwards or Maris Pipers,
and follow the method above.

≈

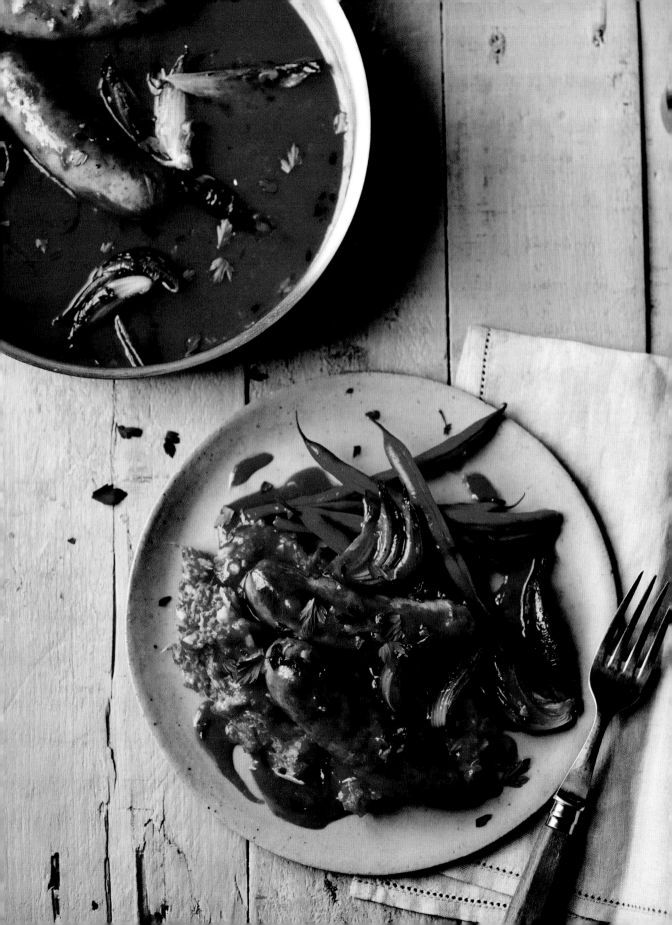

≈ STEAK AND CHIMICHURRI SAUCE ≈

A great treat for a Friday night, this dish is served with chimichurri sauce – a tangy Argentinian favourite, which adds freshness and zing to steak. The sauce can be made in advance if you are short of time. It's great with the chicken on page 102 too.

SERVES 2

562 CALORIES PER SERVING

2 small sweet potatoes (about 300g), chopped

2 x 125g minute steaks, trimmed of any fat

1 tsp olive oil

salt and freshly ground black pepper

CHIMICHURRI SAUCE

10g parsley

1 small garlic clove

1 shallot, quartered

a good pinch or 2 of chilli flakes

4 sprigs of oregano, leaves picked off (or ½ tsp dried oregano)

4 tbsp extra virgin olive oil

2 tbsp red wine vinegar

1 First make the sauce. Put all the ingredients into a small blender. Add a tablespoon of water and blitz until the herbs, garlic and shallot are finely chopped and the mixture has blended to make a sauce. Season the sauce well and set it aside.

2 Put the sweet potatoes into a saucepan and cover them with cold water. Put a lid on the pan and bring the water to the boil, then simmer for 12 minutes until the potatoes are just tender. Drain the potatoes, season and mash them well, then keep the mash warm until you're ready to serve.

3 Meanwhile, cook the steaks. Heat a griddle pan over a medium heat until hot. Brush the steaks with oil and season them well. When the pan is hot, add the steaks and cook them for about 1 minute on each side. Set the steaks aside on a board, covered, for a couple of minutes to rest.

4 Slice the steaks into thin strips and serve with the sweet potato mash and some salad. Scrape any juices from the rested steak over each plate and drizzle a tablespoon of sauce on top.

CREAMY SPINACH

For an extra treat, make some creamy spinach. Put 200g of spinach in a separate pan with 2 tablespoons of cold water. Cover and steam until wilted, then drain it well and tip it back into the pan. Season, then stir in a tablespoon of crème fraiche and 5g of grated Parmesan cheese.

TOM'S TIP

The chimichurri sauce will keep for up to a week in the fridge in a sealed container or a clean jam jar.

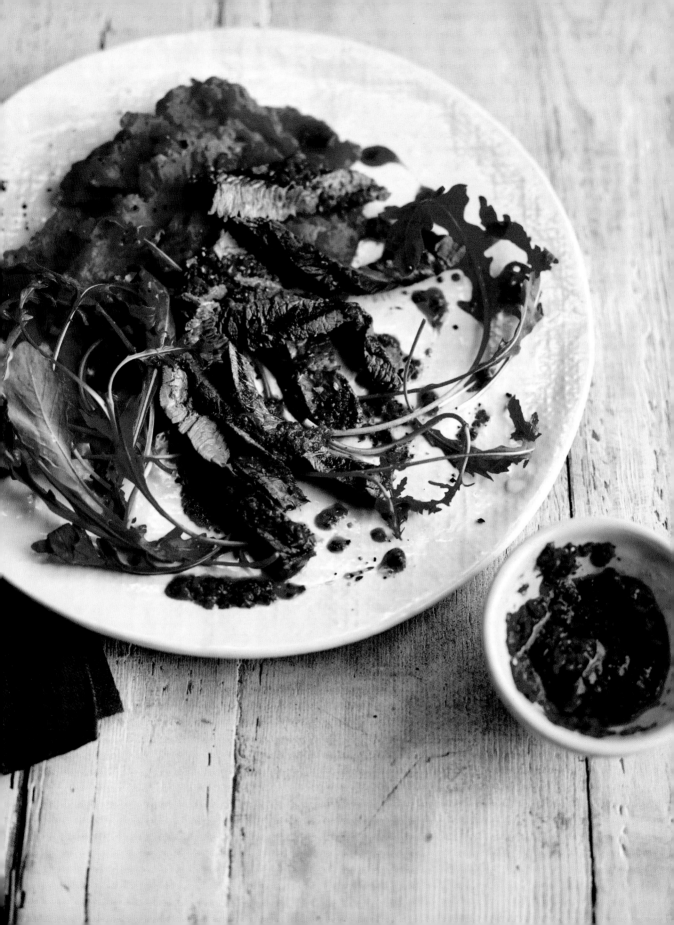

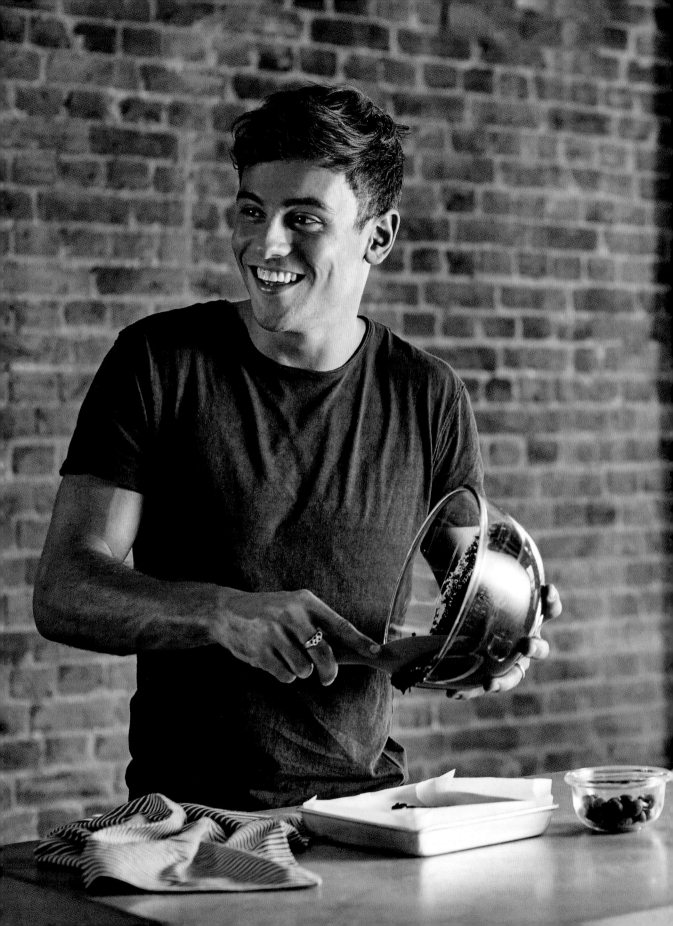

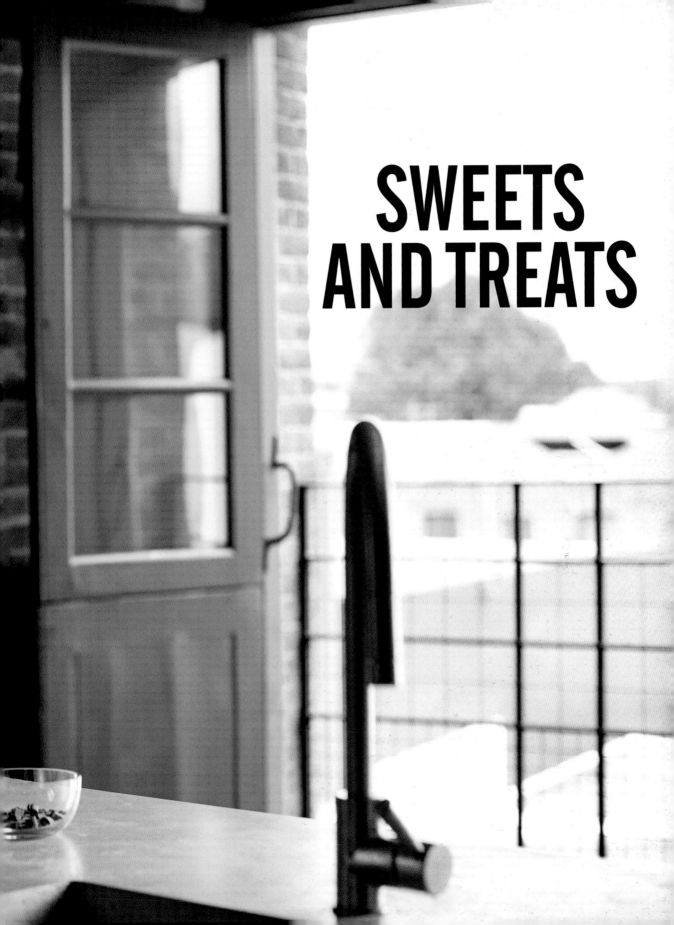

SWEETS
AND TREATS

≈ HOT CHEESECAKES ≈
WITH A NAUGHTY TOPPING

Cheesecake is my all-time favourite dessert – I just love it and will eat any kind.
The great thing about these mini versions is that you only have one portion, rather
than cutting into a large cheesecake and having a massive slice – then another!

SERVES 2

474 CALORIES PER SERVING

45g walnut digestives (see p. 153) or use 45g ready-made digestives

20g melted butter

1 large egg, separated

115g full-fat cream cheese

1 tbsp runny honey

1 tsp cornflour

1 tsp vanilla extract

TOPPING

fresh raspberries, 28g Daim bar, smashed, or 15g dark chocolate

1 Preheat the oven to 170°C/150°C Fan/ Gas 3. Whizz the digestive biscuits in a mini food processor to make fine crumbs. Tip them into a bowl, then stir in the melted butter and mix well. Divide the mixture between 2 x 150ml ramekins.

2 Put the egg white in a clean bowl and whisk with an electric hand whisk or a balloon whisk until the egg white just holds its shape. The balloon whisk takes a little longer than the electric but it's great upper arm exercise!

3 In a separate bowl, whisk the cream cheese, honey, egg yolk, cornflour and vanilla extract, using the same whisk – no need to wash it – until smooth.

4 Add a spoonful of the egg white to the cream cheese mixture and fold together. Add the remaining egg white and fold it in until smooth.

5 Divide the cream cheese mixture between the ramekins. Put them on a baking tray and bake them in the oven for 30 minutes until the cheesecake has cooked. Take them out of the oven and leave to cool for 10 minutes before serving.

6 Serve topped with raspberries and pieces of Daim bar or dark chocolate.

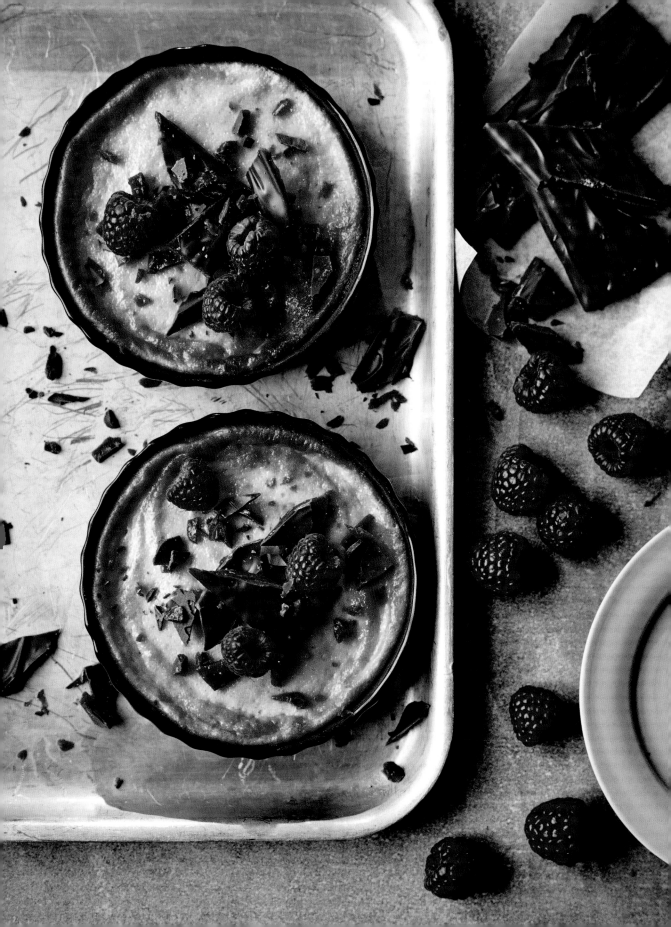

≈ PINEAPPLE CRISP ≈

This tropical treat is super healthy so if you're craving something sweet it will hit the spot without ruining all your hard work. It takes minutes to put together and makes a good light pudding to follow a big meal.

SERVES 2

300 CALORIES PER SERVING

4 thin slices of pineapple, peeled

2 tbsp rolled oats

1 tbsp unsweetened desiccated coconut

1 tbsp pumpkin seeds

2 tsp sunflower seeds

2 tbsp maple syrup

zest of ½ lime

2 tbsp Greek yoghurt, to serve

1 Preheat the oven to 200°C/180°C Fan/ Gas 6.

2 Put the pineapple slices on a baking tray. Sprinkle the rolled oats, coconut, seeds and maple syrup over them, then scatter over the lime zest.

3 Bake the pineapple in the oven for 20 minutes until it's cooked through and the topping is golden. Serve with Greek yoghurt.

TOM'S TIP

This is good for breakfast too, with a spoonful of Greek yoghurt on the side.

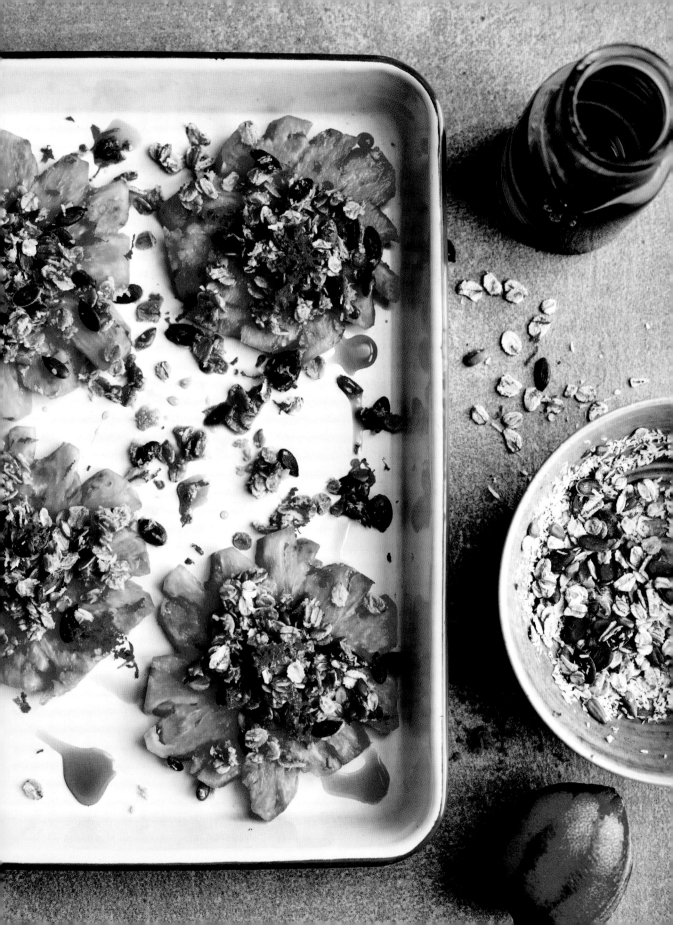

~ WHOLEMEAL CHEESY SCONES ~

These light, savoury scones are a doddle to make and so good to eat.
They're best warm from the oven, but you can keep them in an airtight
container for up to two days, then split and toast them.

MAKES 8 SCONES

193 CALORIES PER SCONE

225g self-raising wholemeal
flour, sifted

50g unsalted butter, cubed

2 tsp linseeds

50g mature Cheddar
cheese, grated

2 tbsp freshly chopped herbs,
such as chives, thyme and
parsley

150ml whole milk

salt

1 Preheat the oven to 220°C/200°C Fan/Gas
7. Line a baking tray with baking paper.

2 Put the flour in a food processor and add
the butter. Whizz a couple of times until
the mixture resembles breadcrumbs. If you
prefer, you can also do this in a bowl by
rubbing the butter in with your fingertips.
Stir in the linseeds, cheese and herbs and
season with a good pinch of salt.

3 If you've used a food processor, tip
the mixture into a bowl. Make a well
in the centre and pour in the milk, then
use a round-bladed knife to stir everything
together to make a rough dough. Add
a splash more milk if the mixture
looks dry.

4 Bring the dough together with your
hands, then tip it gently on to a board
and knead it lightly and quickly until the
dough is smooth. Pat the dough down and
shape it into a round about 2.5cm thick.
Cut the round in half, then cut each half
into 4 wedges.

5 Transfer the wedges to the lined baking
tray and bake for 12–15 minutes, until
just golden. Remove them from the oven
and put them on a wire rack to cool
slightly before eating.

TOM'S TIP
I love to eat these cheesy scones
with a bowl of hot soup, such as
my roasted squash soup (p. 46).
≈

~ WALNUT DIGESTIVE BISCUITS ~

These treats contain much less sugar than shop-bought digestives and are perfect
for a snack when you're running low on energy and need a little something.
Spread them with a slick of cream cheese, cottage cheese or ricotta.

MAKES 20 BISCUITS

70 CALORIES PER BISCUIT

75g softened butter

40g thick honey

pinch of salt

100g wholemeal flour
or rye flour

50g rolled oats, roughly
chopped in a blender

25g walnuts, finely chopped

1 Put the butter, honey and a good pinch of salt into a bowl and beat them together until the mixture looks creamy and smooth. If the butter is soft enough, you can do this with a wooden spoon. Add the flour, oats and walnuts, then continue to work the mixture to make a rough dough.

2 Bring the mixture together with your hands and knead it until smooth. Flatten the dough into a rough round, wrap it in a piece of baking paper and put it in the fridge to chill for 15 minutes. Preheat the oven to 180°C/160°C Fan/Gas 4.

3 Unwrap the dough and roll it out to a thickness of 4–5mm. Stamp out 20 rounds using a 5cm cutter. Prick each round twice with a fork and put them on a baking tray.

4 Bake the biscuits in the oven for 12–15 minutes until they're golden, turning the baking tray around half way through to ensure the colour is even. Transfer the biscuits to a wire rack to cool, then store them in an airtight container for up to 3 days.

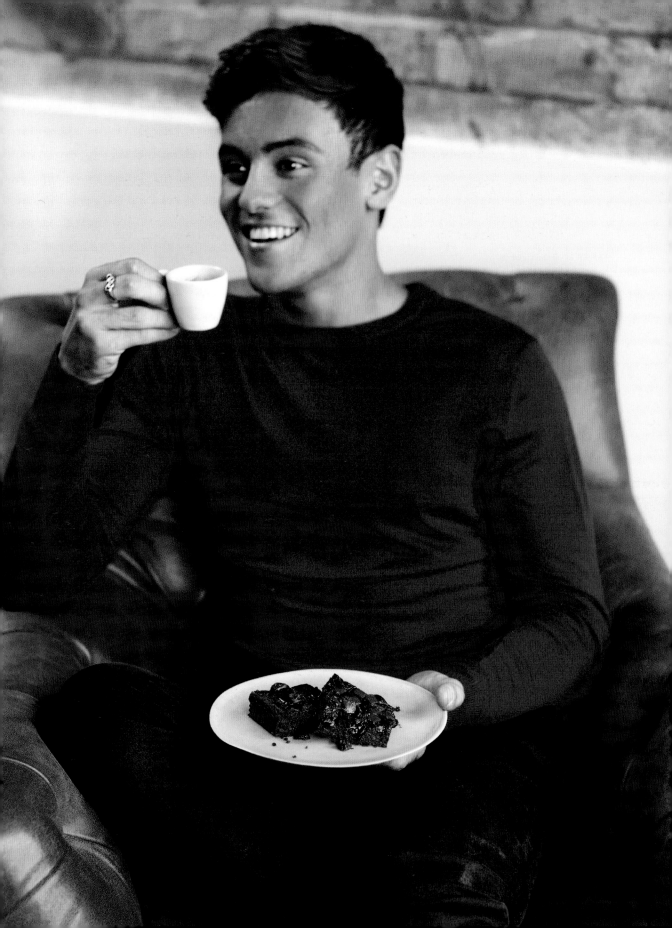

NOT-SO-NAUGHTY
~ CHOCOLATE BROWNIES ~

I am a real sucker for a good brownie and this recipe is awesome – and lower in sugar than most. These brownies contain oats and ground almonds instead of flour so the texture is slightly different from normal, but they are perfect when you just have to have something sweet. If you like your brownies squidgy, bake them for just 15 minutes instead of 18.

MAKES 25 SQUARES

56 CALORIES PER SQUARE

50g each of dried prunes and dates

1 tsp vanilla extract

40g cocoa

35g rolled oats, whizzed in a blender until fine

30g ground almonds

2 medium eggs

1 tsp baking powder

75g unrefined light soft brown sugar

100g Greek yoghurt

20g dark chocolate chips (70% cocoa solids)

50g blueberries

1 Soak the prunes and dates in 100ml of just-boiled water for half an hour. Preheat the oven to 200°C/180°C Fan/Gas 6. Line a 20cm square baking tin with baking paper.

2 Whizz the prunes, dates and soaking liquor in a food processor to make a purée. Transfer this to a bowl and add the vanilla extract.

3 Add the cocoa, oats, ground almonds, eggs, baking powder, sugar and Greek yoghurt. Whisk everything together with a balloon whisk to make a smooth batter, then scrape the mixture into the prepared baking tin, levelling it out to the corners with a spatula.

4 Sprinkle over the dark chocolate chips and blueberries and bake in the oven for 18 minutes. Leave the brownie in the tin to cool for 10 minutes, then transfer it to a board to cool until warm. Slice into 25 squares and serve.

≈ PEAR AND BLACKBERRY ≈ CRUMBLE

This recipe is easy to cook and is a delicious and comforting treat. Wholemeal flour is less processed and has more fibre than white and the fruit is sweet enough, so you really don't need much sugar. The nuts add a healthy dose of unsaturated fat and vitamins and minerals.

SERVES 2

256 CALORIES PER SERVING

1 small Comice pear, quartered, cored and chopped

about 75g blackberries

juice of ¼ orange

1 tsp ground mixed spice

20g chilled butter

30g wholemeal flour, sifted

20g unrefined light soft brown sugar

10g pecans, finely chopped

1 Preheat the oven to 200°C/180°C Fan/Gas 6. Put the pear, blackberries, orange juice and half the mixed spice in a bowl and mix everything together. Divide the mixture between 2 x 300ml ramekins.

2 In a separate bowl, rub the butter into the flour so it forms little clumps (it shouldn't be as fine as breadcrumbs), then stir in the remaining mixed spice, the sugar and pecans.

3 Spoon the topping on to the fruit, dividing it equally between the ramekins. Bake the crumbles in the oven for 15–20 minutes until they're golden on top and the fruit is soft.

TOM'S TIP

These crumbles are also good made with apples and blackberries or with plums or apricots – whatever is in season.

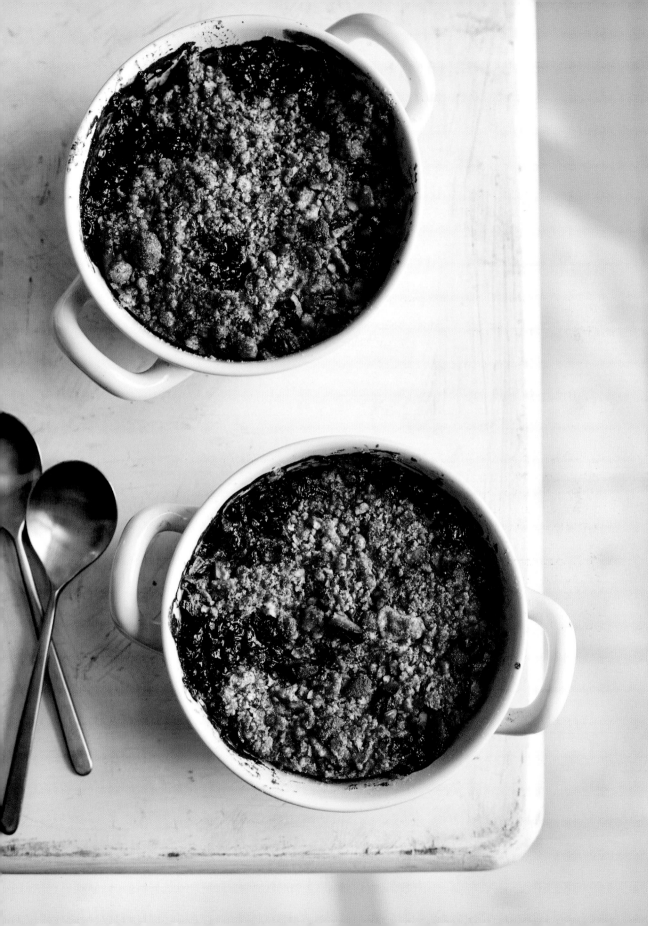

≈ STICKY TOFFEE PUDDINGS ≈

Sticky toffee pudding is one of my favourite desserts but it is usually very high in sugar. My healthier version contains very little sugar and mixes plain and wholemeal flour but is still mouth-wateringly good.

SERVES 2

346 CALORIES PER SERVING

35g butter, softened, plus extra for greasing

50g dates, chopped

¼ tsp bicarbonate of soda

25g unrefined light soft brown sugar

1 medium egg

25g plain flour

25g wholemeal flour

½ tsp baking powder

plain yoghurt, to serve (optional)

1 Grease 2 x 150ml ramekins and line the bases with baking paper. Preheat the oven to 200°C/180°C Fan/Gas 4.

2 Put the dates in a bowl and add the bicarbonate of soda and 75ml of just-boiled water. Set the dates aside for 30 minutes to soak.

3 Beat the 35g of butter and the sugar together in a small bowl. Add the egg, then fold in both types of flour and the baking powder. Fold in the date mixture.

4 Spoon the mixture into the ramekins and bake the puddings in the oven for 20–25 minutes until they've risen and are golden on top. You can check that they are done by pushing a skewer into the centre – it should come out clean. Turn them out and serve with a spoonful of plain yoghurt.

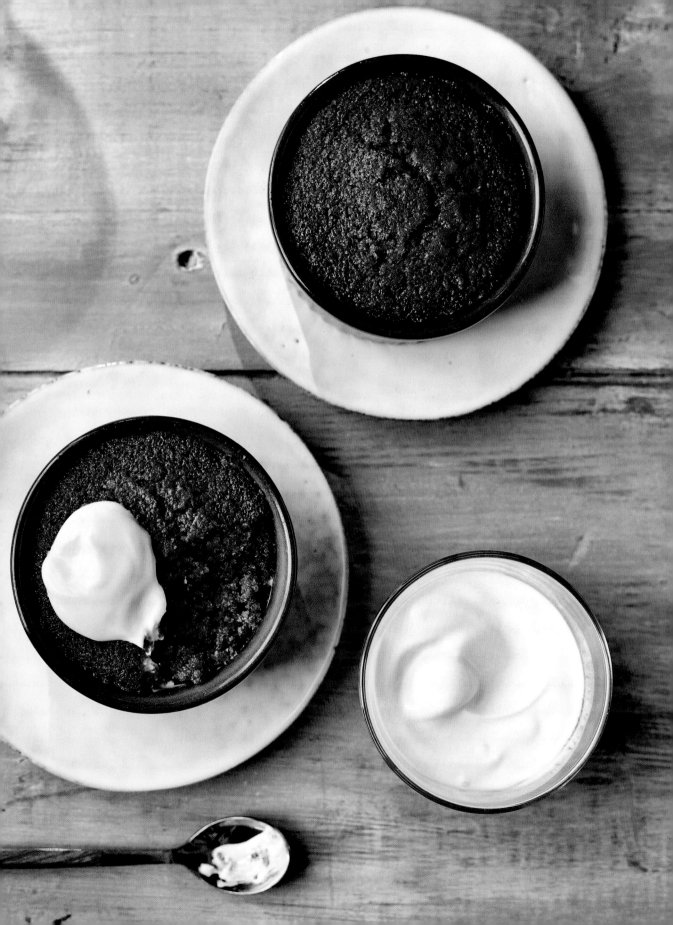

∼ HOT RASPBERRY PUDDINGS ∼

Berries are a great source of antioxidants and vitamin C, so these cute
little puds deliver on nutrition and flavour! Serve them in their pots or turn
them out on to plates and serve with some extra berries if you like.

SERVES 2

428 CALORIES PER SERVING

100g raspberries, plus extra
for serving

1 medium egg

40g thick-set honey or
unrefined golden caster sugar

50g self-raising
wholemeal flour

50g whole almonds

½ tsp baking powder

2 tsp olive oil

10g flaked almonds

1 Preheat the oven to 200°C/180°C Fan/
Gas 6. Divide the raspberries between
2 x 150ml ovenproof pots or ramekins.

2 Put the egg in a bowl and add the honey
or sugar. Whisk with an electric hand
whisk until the mixture is thick and
moussey – this will take about 5 minutes.
You can do this with a balloon whisk but
it will take longer (about twice the time)
although it's great exercise for your upper
arm muscles!

3 Whizz the flour and almonds together
in a food processor until fine and add
the baking powder.

4 Spoon the flour mixture on top of the
egg mixture, then carefully pour the
olive oil around the outside. Fold everything
together with a large metal spoon. It will
drop in volume, but don't worry, this is fine.

5 Divide the mixture evenly between the
pots and scatter the flaked almonds on
top. Bake the puddings in the oven for about
20 minutes until the sponge is golden and
a skewer inserted into the centre comes out
clean. Serve the puddings in the pots or
turn them out. Enjoy while hot.

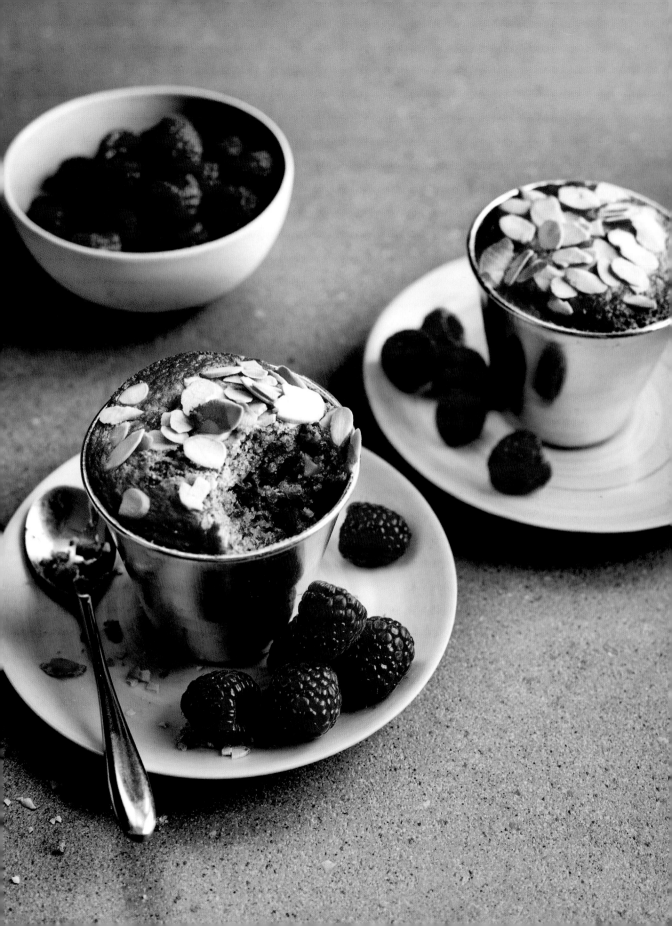

⪞ BANOFFEE PIE ⪞

This luxurious dessert is deliciously crunchy and creamy and a healthier alternative to the classic recipe, which is one of my all-time favourites. It's raw, gluten-free and free of refined sugar – just what you need to curb those cravings.

SERVES 2

364 CALORIES PER SERVING

30g dates

20g cashew nuts

25g oats

1 tsp coconut oil

2 tsp unsweetened desiccated coconut

zest and juice of ½ lime

1 banana (about 120g), thinly sliced

50g cream cheese

75g Greek yoghurt

2 tsp maple syrup

good pinch of cinnamon (optional)

5g dark chocolate, chopped into thin shavings

1 Put the dates and cashew nuts in a small bowl and pour over enough just-boiled water to cover them. Leave them to soak for 10 minutes.

2 Drain the dates and cashew nuts and put them in a mini food processor with the oats, coconut oil, desiccated coconut and lime zest and whizz to finely chop the ingredients and until it forms a sticky mixture. Spoon the mixture into 2 glasses and push the mixture down with your fingers. Chill for 15 minutes.

3 After 15 minutes, divide the slices of banana between the glasses and add half the lime juice to each. Mix the cream cheese, yoghurt, a teaspoon of maple syrup, the cinnamon, if using, and a tablespoon of cold water together in a bowl and spoon this mixture over the banana slices.

4 To serve, drizzle half a teaspoon of maple syrup over each serving and sprinkle with the chocolate.

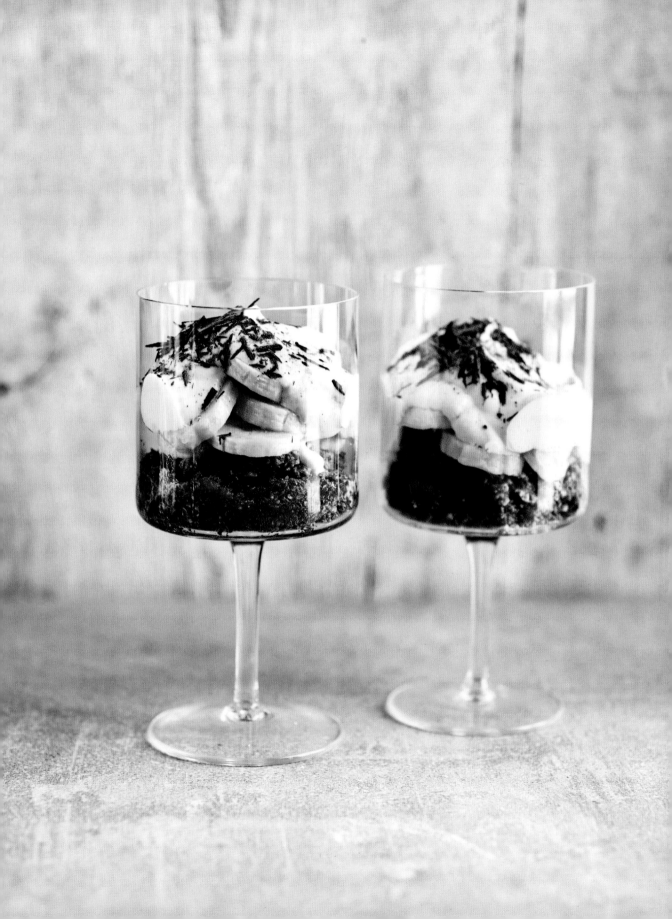

≈ FROZEN YOGHURT ≈

I've always loved ice cream – my friends even bought me an ice cream maker when I was 14! The great thing about this frozen yoghurt is that it is less calorific than normal ice cream but just as delicious. It's sweetened with a little maple syrup and no sugar – so will satisfy your cravings, with none of the guilt. Try the basic recipe, then some of my variations below.

EACH RECIPE MAKES ENOUGH FOR 6 SERVINGS

92 CALORIES PER SERVING

500ml natural yoghurt

3–4 tbsp maple syrup

2 tsp vanilla extract

1 Put the yoghurt, maple syrup and vanilla extract into an ice cream maker and churn until frozen. Transfer the mixture to a freezer-proof container and eat within a month.

2 If you don't have an ice cream maker, put the mixture into a freezer-proof container and whisk with a balloon whisk every 20–30 minutes until frozen.

VARIATIONS

Here are some variations. For an extra treat, the mango and lime is delicious with some passion fruit juice and seeds spooned over the top. Try the chocolate and orange with a handful of raspberries, and scatter a few extra toasted chopped peanuts over the peanut butter and banana version.

MANGO AND LIME

113 CALORIES PER SERVING

Whizz 200g of chopped mango (the flesh of about 1 medium mango) and the zest of half a lime in a food processor to make a smooth purée. Stir this into the yoghurt mixture above and freeze in an ice cream maker.

CHOCOLATE AND ORANGE

112 CALORIES PER SERVING

Stir 20g of cocoa powder, the zest of quarter of an orange and 1 tablespoon of maple syrup into the yoghurt mixture above and churn. The cocoa is quite bitter, which is why it needs an extra spoonful of maple syrup to soften it.

PEANUT BUTTER AND BANANA

148 CALORIES PER SERVING

Stir 40g of peanut and almond butter (see p. 172, or use ready-made peanut butter) and a mashed banana (about 100g) into the yoghurt mixture above and churn.

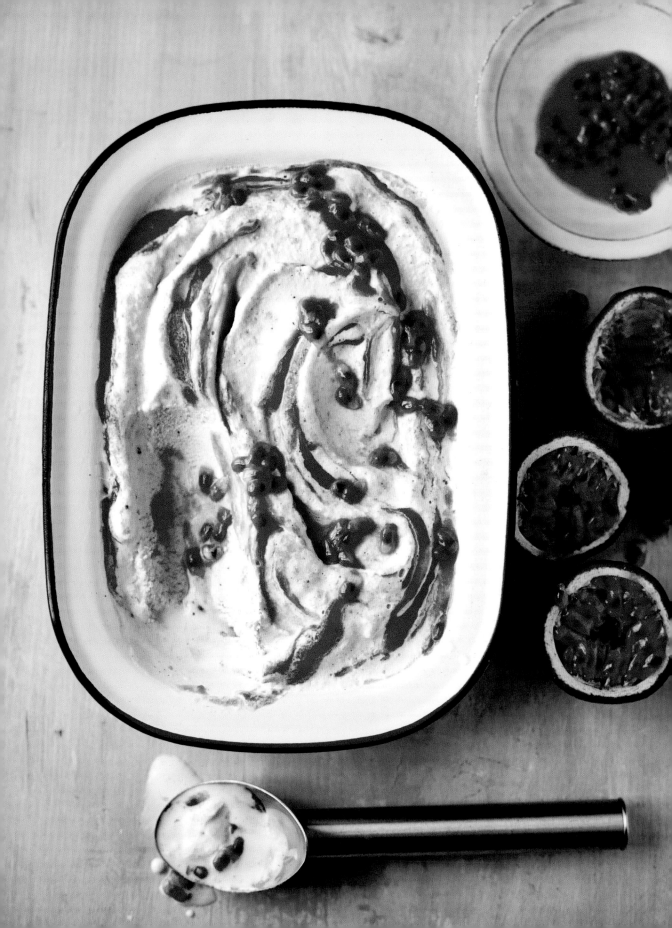

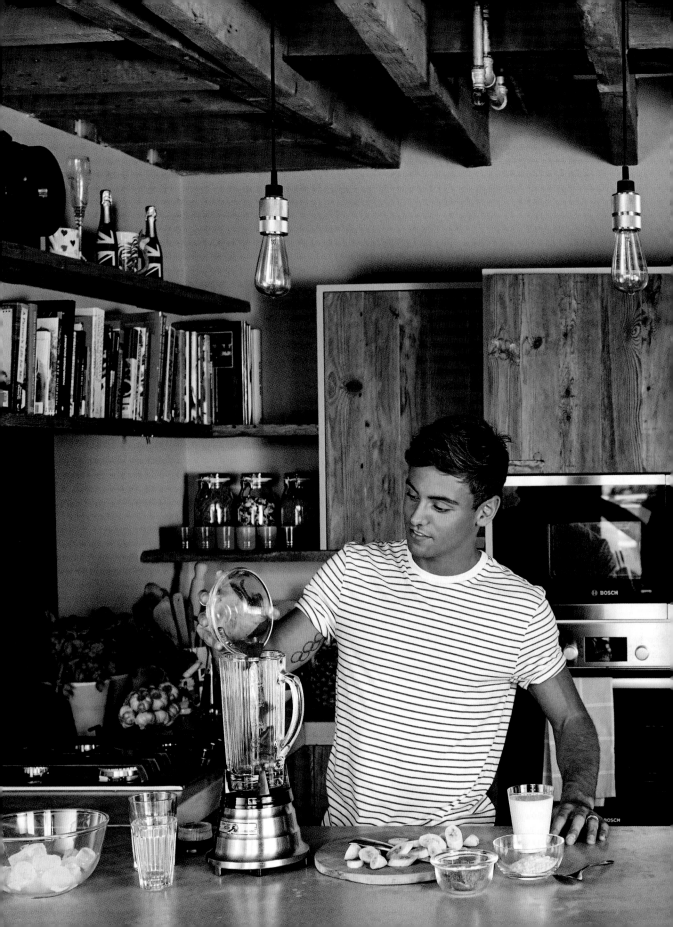

SNACKS AND DRINKS

≈ PICK-ME-UP POWER BALLS ≈

Instead of buying sugar-frosted, expensive and preservative-packed protein bars
whizz up some of these delicious combos of dried fruit and nuts instead. Ideal for
a post workout, these have none of the junk and plenty of protein, thanks to their
energy-boosting ingredients. BTW, ground coffee might sound odd but it goes
really well with the dates and nuts and enriches their flavour. And the chilli
in the almond and choc version adds warmth and a little kick!

**EACH RECIPE MAKES
10 POWER BALLS**

**DATE AND PECAN
POWER BALLS**

47 CALORIES PER BALL

100g dates

20g flaked almonds

30g pecans

2 pinches of ground coffee

**TROPICAL FRUIT
POWER BALLS**

47 CALORIES PER BALL

20g unsweetened dried mango

30g unsweetened dried
pineapple

50g dried apricots

30g whole cashew nuts

2 tsp unsweetened
coconut flakes

**PEANUT BUTTER AND
MANGO POWER BALLS**

37 CALORIES PER BALL

50g dried mango pieces

25g peanut butter (ready-made
or see p. 172)

50g apricots

¼ tsp ground cinnamon

**ALMOND AND CHOCOLATE
POWER BALLS**

41 CALORIES PER BALL

50g dates

50g whole almonds

1 tsp cocoa nibs

2 generous pinches of
chilli flakes

1 All the power balls are made in the same
way. Put the ingredients for the variation
you are making into a small food processor
with a teaspoon of just-boiled water and
pulse until smooth. Take out a piece of the
mixture with your fingers and squeeze it.
It's ready when it sticks together well.

2 Scrape the mixture out on to a board
and divide it into 10 even pieces. Roll
each piece into a ball and put it on a plate.
Chill in the fridge until firm. You can freeze
these little goodies in an airtight container
for up to a month or store them in the
fridge for a week.

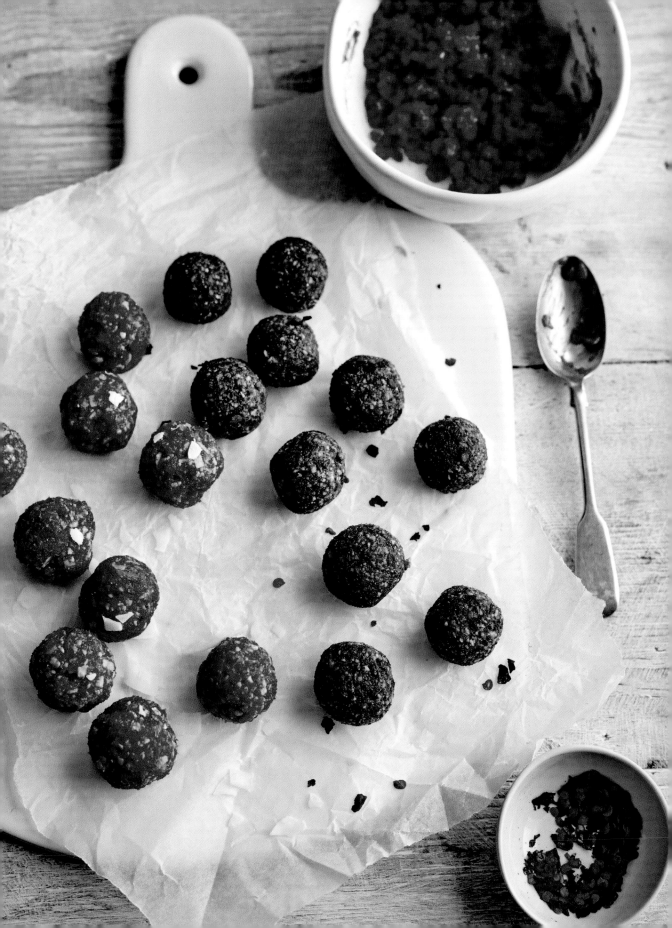

~ BANANA AND PECAN MUFFINS ~

If you're mad about bananas – like me – these muffins are a real treat. There's no refined sugar in them, just a smidgen of honey to bring out the sweetness of the bananas. Make sure you choose really ripe fruit – when there are a few black spots on the skin, bananas are very sweet and just right for this recipe.

MAKES 8

262 CALORIES PER MUFFIN

200g wholemeal flour

2 tsp baking powder

50g sultanas

25g pecan nuts, chopped

300g ripe bananas, peeled

25g honey

100g Greek yoghurt

100ml whole milk

1 medium egg

60g butter, melted and cooled for 5 minutes

1 Preheat the oven to 200°C/Fan 180°C/Gas 6. Line a muffin tin with 8 paper muffin cases.

2 Put the flour, baking powder, sultanas and pecan nuts in a bowl and stir everything together.

3 In a separate bowl, mash the bananas and honey together until smooth. Stir in the Greek yoghurt, milk and egg.

4 Add the wet mixture to the flour mixture, then pour the melted butter over the top. Using a large metal spoon, fold everything together quickly until the ingredients are roughly mixed. There should still be a few floury patches and the mixture will look claggy, but don't worry – it's meant to be like that. The secret to light muffins is to have a light touch and not to fold the mixture together until completely smooth.

5 Divide the mixture between the muffin cases. Bake the muffins in the oven for 20–25 minutes until they're nicely risen and golden on top and a skewer inserted into the centre comes out clean. Remove the muffins from the tin and leave them to cool on a wire rack until just warm before eating.

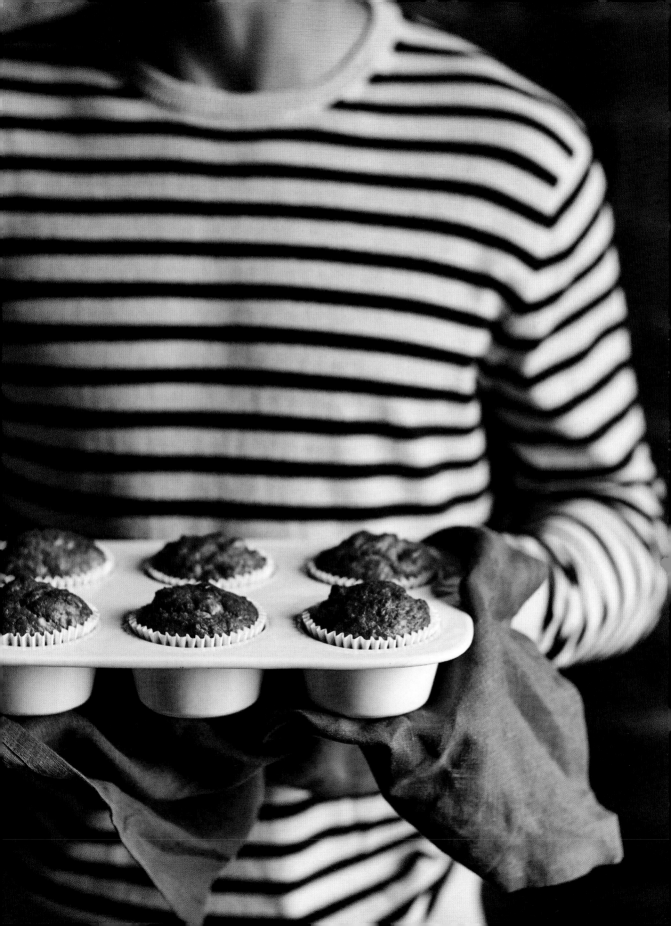

≈ PEANUT BUTTER ≈
THREE WAYS

Nut butters combine fibre, heart-healthy monounsaturated fat and protein, meaning they help you feel fuller for longer. They're packed with vitamins and minerals but they're also high in calories so be sure to watch your portions. All of these can be stored in the cupboard for one month.

PEANUT AND COCONUT BUTTER

MAKES ABOUT 225G

100 CALORIES PER TBSP (15G)

200g peanuts

25g unsweetened desiccated coconut

20g coconut oil

good pinch of sea salt

Put the peanuts, coconut, coconut oil and salt into a food processor and whizz for 5–10 minutes until the mixture is smooth and butter-like. Spoon into a clean, sterilised jar and seal. Great on an oatcake.

PEANUT AND CASHEW NUT BUTTER

MAKES ABOUT 200G

90 CALORIES PER TBSP (15G)

100g peanuts

100g cashews

good pinch of sea salt

1 Put the peanuts and cashews into a large frying pan and place the pan over a low heat. Cook, tossing the nuts every now and then, for about 5–10 minutes until golden.

2 Tip the nuts into a food processor and add the salt. Whizz for 10–20 minutes, scraping down the side of the bowl occasionally, until the mixture is smooth and butter-like. Spoon into a clean, sterilised jar and seal. Lovely on porridge with a splash of milk.

PEANUT AND ALMOND BUTTER

MAKES ABOUT 200G

93 CALORIES PER TBSP (15G)

100g peanuts

100g almonds

½ tsp ground mixed spice

½ tsp ground cinnamon

good pinch of sea salt

1 Put the peanuts and almonds into a large frying pan and place the pan over a low heat. Cook, tossing the nuts every now and then, for about 5–10 minutes until golden.

2 Tip the nuts into a food processor and add the spices and salt. Whizz for 10–20 minutes, scraping down the side of the bowl occasionally, until the mixture is smooth. Spoon into a clean, sterilised jar and seal. Good with porridge or on toast.

≋ TOM'S CHOCOLATE ≋
AND HAZELNUT SPREAD

This is my awesome version of a much-loved chocolate spread. It's very indulgent, so shouldn't be eaten very often but if you are craving something sweet and have worked hard – enjoy! Serve a small spoonful spread on slices of banana. You do need a good food processor with sharp blades to mix this up properly.

MAKES ABOUT 300G – ENOUGH TO FILL 1 LARGE JAR

95 CALORIES PER TBSP (15G)

200g whole hazelnuts in their skins

2 tbsp sunflower oil or light olive oil

15g cacao or cocoa powder

3 tbsp honey

25g dark chocolate (at least 80% cocoa solids)

½ tsp ground cinnamon

1 Put the hazelnuts in a frying pan. Heat them gently over a medium heat for 2–3 minutes, tossing them every now and then, until the nuts are toasted and the skins are starting to blister. Take care not to overcook the nuts or let the skin burn or the spread will taste bitter.

2 Take the pan off the heat and tip the nuts into a food processor. Add the oil, cacao or cocoa powder, honey, dark chocolate and cinnamon and whizz until the mixture is smooth. This will take a while, so stop the machine every now and then and scrape the mixture down the sides of the bowl with a rubber spatula.

3 When the mixture is nice and smooth, spoon it into a sterilised jar and seal with a lid. The spread keeps well in a cupboard for up to a month.

TOM'S TIP
This is my mum's quick way of sterilising jars. Wash the jars and lids in soapy water and rinse well. Stand them in the sink and pour just-boiled water into the jars and lids so that the water flows over the sides. Leave them for a couple of minutes, then tip the water away. Be careful, the jars will be hot!
≋

QUICK
≈ PROTEIN SHAKES ≈

Protein shakes are great after a workout to help recover your strength and restore nutrients. These are a few of my favourites but you can experiment with other flavours too. Use really ripe bananas for a good strong flavour.

SERVES 2

171 CALORIES PER SHAKE

175ml almond milk or whole milk

1 banana, sliced

1 tbsp peanut butter

2 tbsp protein powder

2 ice cubes

1 tsp vanilla extract

1 Put all the ingredients into a blender and whizz until smooth. If your blender has a tendency to leak, wrap a tea towel round the edge of it and hold it down tightly while it blitzes the ingredients together.

2 Divide the mixture between 2 glasses and serve.

VARIATIONS

STRAWBERRY

181 CALORIES PER SHAKE

Add 50g of hulled, chopped strawberries in place of the vanilla extract and swap the peanut butter for almond butter.

CHOCOLATE

236 CALORIES PER SHAKE

Add 2 tablespoons of cocoa or cacao powder in place of the vanilla extract and swap the peanut butter for almond butter. Add a teaspoon of maple syrup or honey too, as the cocoa/cacao can taste quite bitter.

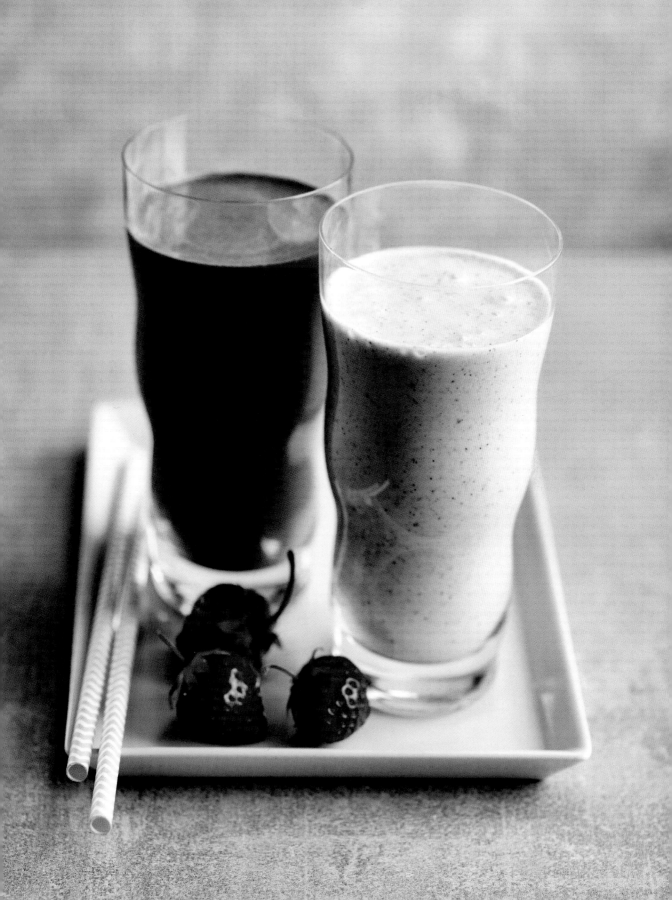

MY DAILY WORKOUTS

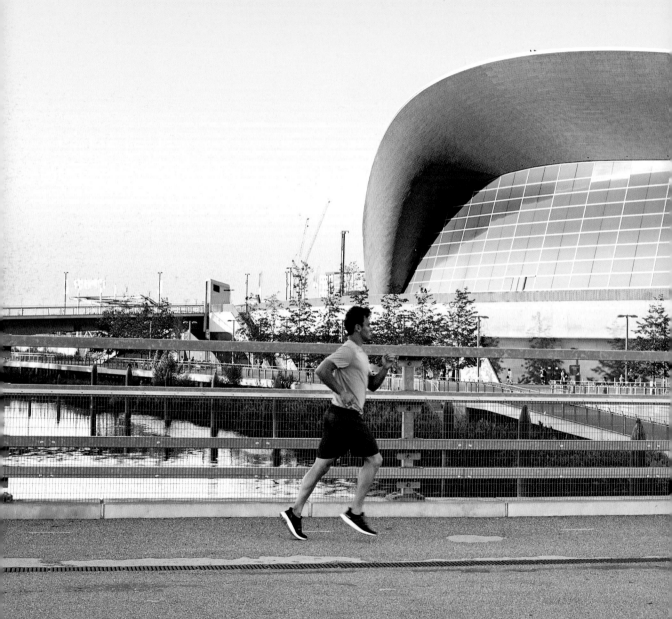

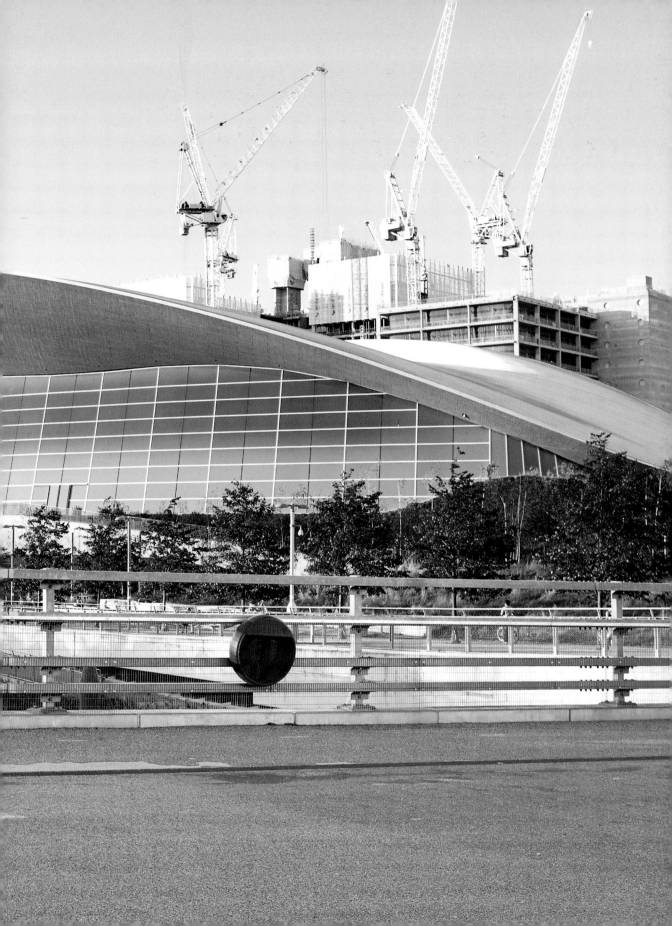

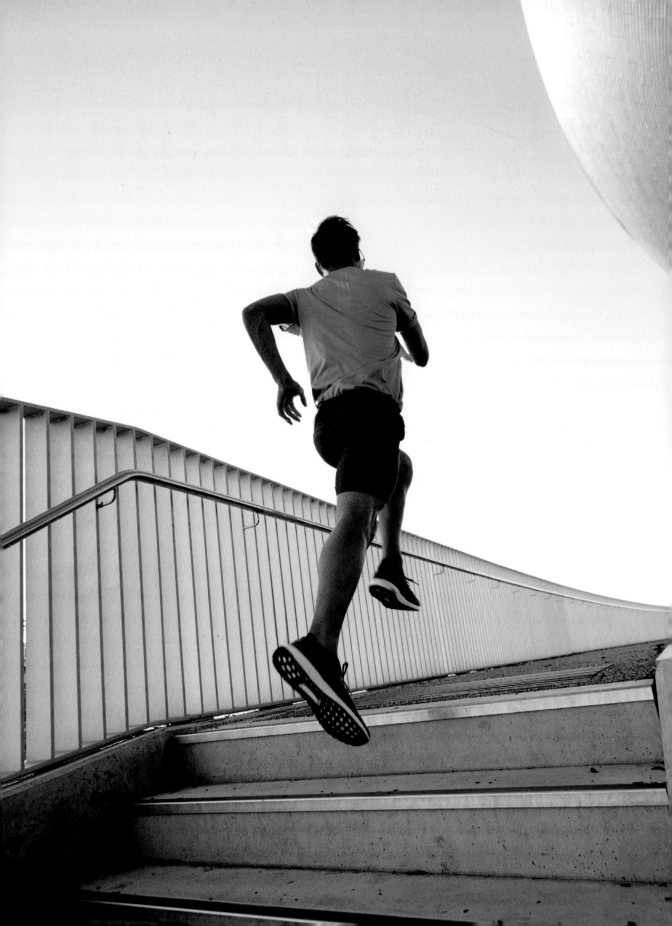

≈ GET MOVING! ≈

Exercise is my life. When I'm training, I exercise for five hours a day, six days a week –
and I know that's not for everybody! But it's so important to do what you can. Just
20 minutes of high-intensity exercise, five days a week, will help you get fit, tone up
and improve your health. It's totally worth it and you don't need an expensive
gym membership or any specialist equipment.

MY HOME WORKOUTS

My 20-minute routines are simple, effective
and fun, and they're designed to build strength
and lose unwanted pounds. You can also
adapt them to be more challenging as your
fitness improves. They're based on high-
intensity interval training (HIIT), which
describes any workout that alternates between
intense bursts of activity and fixed periods
of less intense activity. It's the most effective
way to burn calories in a short amount
of time. What's more, HIIT boosts your
metabolism and increases your endurance.
You're more likely to stick with it and it's
great for your heart. Best of all – you can
do these workouts anywhere, at any time!

FIND YOUR OWN PACE

If you're new to exercise routines, the key
to success is doing the correct moves at
your own pace – don't rush things at first.
My mum ran the London Marathon in 2012,
then the Plymouth half-marathon in 2014
and I encouraged her to build up her fitness
slowly and steadily. She trained with a group
of other women and found it really helpful.
It's always good to have a friend to train with.

BUILD FITNESS INTO YOUR LIFE

Build fitness into your life as and where
you can: walk to work or to and from the
shops, do some star jumps during the ad
breaks when you're watching the telly or
go on family bike rides – every little helps.
Let everyone know what you are doing and
get them to support you. While my mum
was training, my brothers and I often
cycled along with her, shouting words
of encouragement!

LISTEN TO YOUR BODY

Always listen to your body. Push yourself
as much as you can, but modify the moves
if you need to and always focus on your
technique. Be sure to warm up before
you start the routines, then cool down
afterwards and do some gentle stretches.

THE ROUTINES

On the following pages you'll find five home
workout routines. Read through the exercises
carefully and practise each one before you
start the routines. Begin with the beginners
version you'll find in the column headed
repetitions and work up to the intermediate
and advanced when you're ready.

FITNESS LIFE HACKS
≈ MYTH BUSTING ≈

We're constantly being bombarded with ideas and quick fixes for keeping to a healthy weight, but do all these things actually work? I have to say that most do not. Here are five commonly held beliefs about diet, exercise and weight loss that are just plain wrong and are a waste of your time!

SKIPPING MEALS WILL HELP YOU LOSE WEIGHT
WRONG

Studies have consistently shown that people who skip meals are heavier than those who don't, because missing food just make you overeat later on. When you skip a meal your body goes into starvation mode and stores calories as fat. Eat regularly to make sure your blood sugar levels stay stable and you don't crave sweet snacks.

NEVER SNACK BETWEEN MEALS
WRONG

Mindless snacking will sabotage any efforts you make to lose weight, but regular healthy snacks are an excellent way of keeping you feeling satisfied between meals. Post-exercise snacks are good for nourishing and repairing your body and then you're less likely to overeat at mealtimes. If you're hungry, pay attention to what your body is telling you.

NEVER EAT FAST FOOD
WRONG

Sometimes we all find ourselves in situations where we need to eat something on the go. Fast food shouldn't be a regular habit, but once in a while, if you choose well, it'll do you no harm. Always choose grilled over fried food, scrape away or avoid ketchup and mayo, and go for a side salad instead of fries. Even cheap fast food restaurants offer a few healthier choices.

AVOID CARBOHYDRATES
WRONG

Many dieters follow low-carb plans, but carbohydrates are an important food group when eaten in the right quantities and as part of a balanced diet. Eat wholegrain carbohydrates, like brown rice and pasta, and avoid refined white carbs.

IF YOU EXERCISE, YOU CAN EAT WHATEVER YOU WANT
WRONG

I so wish this was true but you can never out-exercise a bad diet. To keep your weight stable, have a healthy varied diet, don't overeat, and take regular exercise.

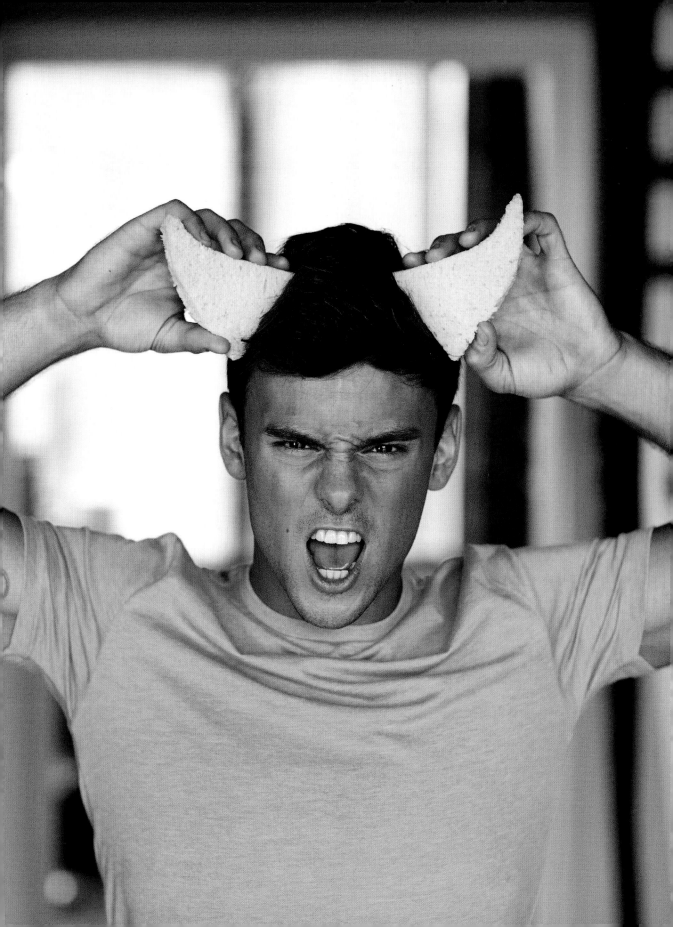

FITNESS LIFE HACKS
≋ BE POSITIVE – IT REALLY WORKS ≋

You've been on holiday and put on a few pounds or you seem to have skipped your exercise routine for a few days. You panic, feel a failure and get drawn into a cycle of negative thinking – it happens to us all and you just need to pick yourself up and think positively again. Here are my tips to help you cope with these moments.

RECOGNISE YOUR NEGATIVE THOUGHTS

Don't let them take you over. Negative thought patterns are repetitive and destructive and they have a direct link to negative emotions. Once you learn to recognise them, you have a choice over how to react. Over time, it becomes easier to recognise the thoughts but then let them wash over you. Say to yourself: 'Okay, that was bad but I can do something about it.'

BE POSITIVE

When you catch yourself worrying or thinking negatively, do something positive and uplifting. For me, this might be going for a good long walk or a run, watching some funny YouTube clips or having a relaxing bath.

DON'T DWELL ON MISTAKES

Remember that no one's perfect. The only thing you can do is move forward, so put whatever is worrying you behind you and move on or start again.

SURROUND YOURSELF WITH POSITIVE PEOPLE

When you're caught up in negative moments, surrounding yourself with or talking to positive people can make a real difference.

STOP COMPARING YOURSELF WITH OTHERS

With social media and TV, it is all too easy to compare ourselves with others. If you notice yourself doing this, stop and deliberately reset your mind. You are you and you're very special.

WHEN YOU CATCH YOURSELF WORRYING,
DO SOMETHING POSITIVE AND UPLIFTING

FITNESS LIFE HACKS
≈ BEING THE BEST POSSIBLE YOU ≈

Are you aiming to get stronger, fitter, leaner? That's great! Whether you're an athlete or not, everyone has a different approach to getting the best from themselves. Here are some tips that have worked for me.

MIX UP YOUR WORKOUTS

The reason I've included different workouts in my routines is because sticking to the same workout over and over again won't give you the best results. As your strength and endurance grows, try to push yourself even harder.

MAKE NOTES ABOUT YOUR PERFORMANCE

Did you do something a bit quicker today? Did you find your workout a bit easier? Keep track of your performance and how much you have improved. This will encourage you and also give you an idea of what improvements to aim for.

TAKE AN ALL-ROUND APPROACH

Wanting to improve your exercise performance is one thing, but it's equally important to think about how you approach your food, rest time and nutrition. By doing this, you will maximise your potential to the fullest.

BUDDY UP

Working out with a friend or family member creates a competitive environment and makes you accountable to someone else besides yourself. Makes it harder to skip your routine too!

DRINK ENOUGH WATER

It's essential to drink enough water when you are exercising. Even mild dehydration affects your physical and mental performance.

AS YOUR STRENGTH AND ENDURANCE GROWS, PUSH YOURSELF HARDER

MONDAY: CORE AND CARDIO
20-MINUTE ROUTINE

SEQUENCE

60 SECONDS
HIGH KNEES

30 SECONDS
SIT-UPS

60 SECONDS
HIGH KNEES

30 SECONDS
OBLIQUE CRUNCHES

REPETITIONS

BEGINNERS
Warm up.
Repeat the sequence six times,
resting for 30 seconds to one
minute between each.
Cool down.

INTERMEDIATE
Warm up.
Repeat the sequence twice
Rest for one minute.
Repeat the sequence twice
Rest for one minute.
Repeat the sequence twice
Rest for one minute.
Cool down.

ADVANCED
Warm up.
Repeat the sequence three times
Rest for one minute.
Repeat the sequence three times
Rest for one minute.
Cool down.

CORE AND CARDIO

HERE'S WHAT TO DO

Read through each exercise and check out the pictures. Start your routine with a warm-up: jog or march on the spot for 30 seconds; follow this with 30 seconds of arm swings, 30 seconds of basic squats, then 30 seconds of shallow lunges.

Follow the routine opposite in the order shown and at the appropriate repetitions level – beginners, intermediate or advanced. Use your mobile phone to time yourself. Finish your routine by walking for a couple of minutes to cool down, then do some stretches.

Let's get started!

HIGH KNEES

1 Run on the spot, while lifting your knees high in the air to a 90-degree angle.

EASIER OPTION

Do this as a walking motion. Make sure that the foot of your raised leg is higher than the knee of your stationary leg.

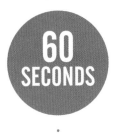

60
SECONDS

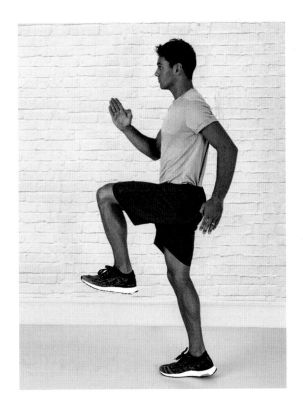

MONDAY: CORE AND CARDIO

SIT-UPS

1 Lie down on your back with your knees bent and your hands behind your ears.

2 Keeping your lower back pressed into the floor, slowly raise your back off the floor. Don't use your hands to pull your neck up, and tuck your neck into your chest as you rise.

3 Come up to a sitting position, then slowly lower yourself down.

TO WORK HARDER

When you're in a sitting position, lift both your legs to a 90-degree angle. Lower them to the floor at the same time as you lower your back to the floor.

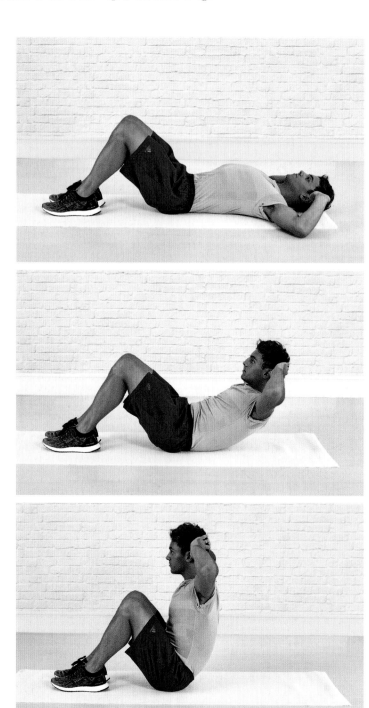

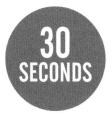

30 SECONDS

REPEAT
60 SECONDS
HIGH KNEES

CORE AND CARDIO

OBLIQUE CRUNCHES

1 Lie on your back, knees bent and feet flat on the floor, hip-width apart.

2 Roll your knees to one side, taking the lower knee to the floor. Place one hand across your body and the other behind your ear.

3 Slowly curl up towards your hips until your lower shoulder is about three inches off the floor. Hold the position, then lower yourself down slowly. Alternate sides with each set.

30 SECONDS

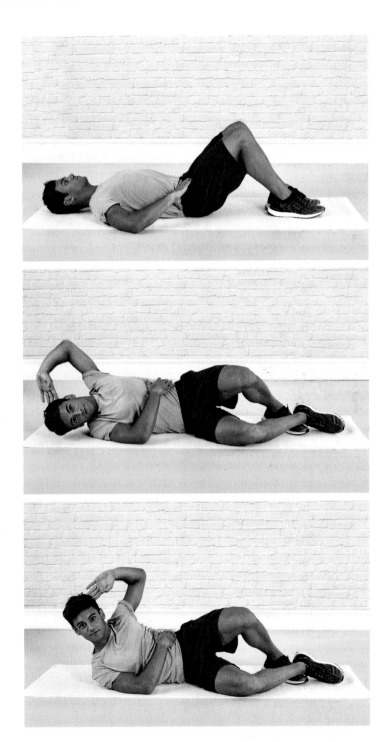

MONDAY: CORE AND CARDIO

COOL DOWN AND STRETCHES

To cool down, walk for two minutes and regulate your breathing. Then stretch the muscles of whatever part of the body you've been working on. Here are some stretches to do after your core and cardio routine.

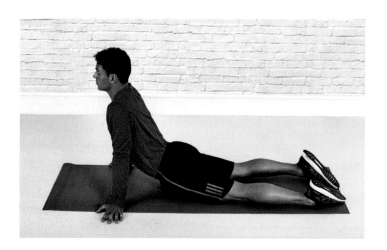

SEAL STRETCH

Lie on your front with your hands under your shoulders. Push up, arching your back and stretching your stomach. Go far enough to feel a good stretch without straining your lower back and hold for 20–30 seconds. Repeat.

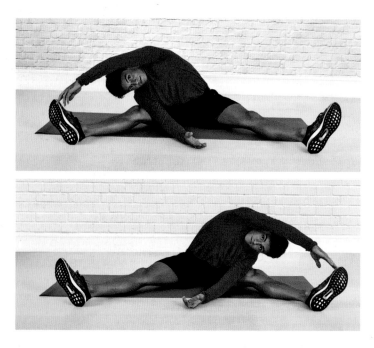

STRADDLE SIDE STRETCH

Sit on the floor with your legs as wide apart as you can manage. Reach your left arm over to your right side to touch your right foot, holding your right arm out in front of you. Hold for 20–30 seconds, then repeat on the other side

TUESDAY: BUTT AND LEG BURNER
20-MINUTE ROUTINE

SEQUENCE

60 SECONDS
JUMPING JACKS

30 SECONDS
SQUATS/SQUAT JUMPS

60 SECONDS
JUMPING JACKS

30 SECONDS
LUNGES

REPETITIONS

BEGINNERS

Warm up.
Repeat the sequence six times,
resting for 30 seconds to one
minute between each.
Cool down.

INTERMEDIATE

Warm up.
Repeat the sequence twice
Rest for one minute.
Repeat the sequence twice
Rest for one minute.
Repeat the sequence twice
Rest for one minute.
Cool down.

ADVANCED

Warm up.
Repeat the sequence three times
Rest for one minute.
Repeat the sequence three times
Rest for one minute.
Cool down.

TUESDAY: BUTT AND LEG BURNER

HERE'S WHAT TO DO

Start with a warm-up: jog or march on the spot for 30 seconds; follow this with 30 seconds of arm swings, 30 seconds of basic squats, then 30 seconds of shallow lunges. Then follow the routine on the previous page at the appropriate repetitions level – beginners, intermediate or advanced.

JUMPING JACKS

1 Stand tall with your arms by your sides and your knees slightly bent.

2 Jump up, extending your arms and legs out into a star shape. Land softly, with your knees together and your hands by your sides. Keep your abs tight and your back straight throughout.

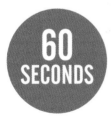

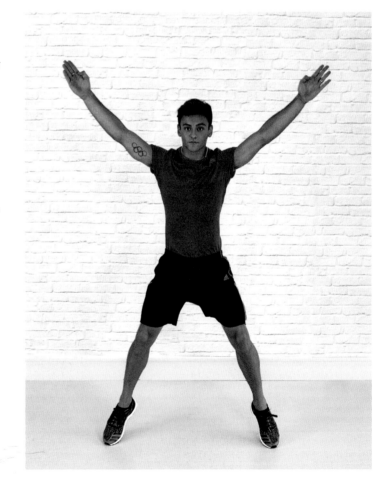

BUTT AND LEG BURNER

SQUATS/SQUAT JUMPS

1 For a basic squat, stand tall with your hands on your hips, legs shoulder-width apart and knees slightly bent.

2 Lower yourself by bending your knees until they are nearly at right angles, with your thighs parallel to the floor. Keep your back straight and do not let your knees extend over your toes. Hold, then return to a standing position.

TO WORK HARDER

Try a squat jump. As you stand up, spring into the air so both feet leave the ground, then land softly, with your hands on your hips.

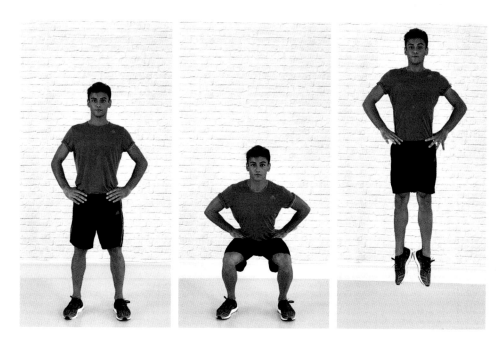

30 SECONDS ..... **REPEAT**
60 SECONDS
JUMPING JACKS

TUESDAY: BUTT AND LEG BURNER

LUNGES

1 Stand tall with your hands on your hips, keeping your core engaged.

2 Move one leg forward and step into a lunge position.

3 Slowly lower your back leg, bringing the front leg as close to a 90-degree angle as possible. Keep your back straight and don't let your knee extend over your toes. Keeping the weight in your heels, push back up to your starting position. Change legs each time you lunge.

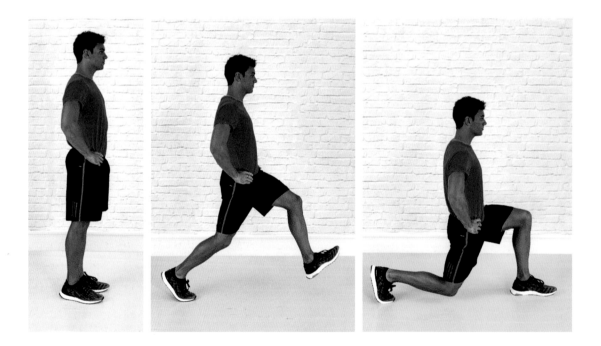

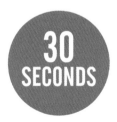

30 SECONDS

BUTT AND LEG BURNER

COOL DOWN AND STRETCHES

To cool down, walk for two minutes and regulate your breathing. Then stretch the muscles of whatever part of the body you've been working on. Here are some stretches to do after your butt and leg burner routine.

GLUTE STRETCH

Sit on the floor with your arms behind you. Extend your left leg, then bend your right leg and put your right foot in line with your left knee. Place your left ankle on your right knee and you should feel a stretch in your glute. Hold for 20–30 seconds, then change legs and repeat.

HIP FLEXOR STRETCH

Stand in a wide split stance. Drop down on to your right knee, keeping your left knee at a right angle and your hips tucked under. Hold for 20–30 seconds, then repeat on the other side. Tighten your glutes for a stronger stretch.

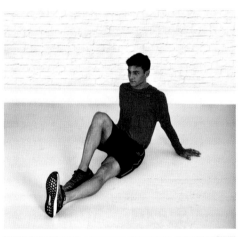

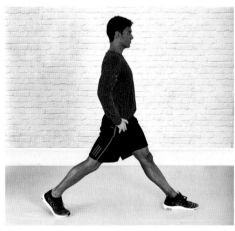

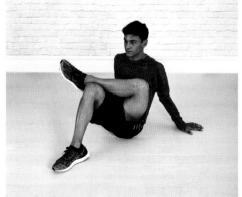

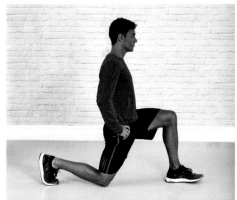

⇌ WEDNESDAY: REST DAY ⇌

A rest day – hurray! Rest days are important to allow
your body to recover from exercise. Try to make sure
you take some light to moderate activity, like going
for a brisk stroll, to keep your muscles loose.

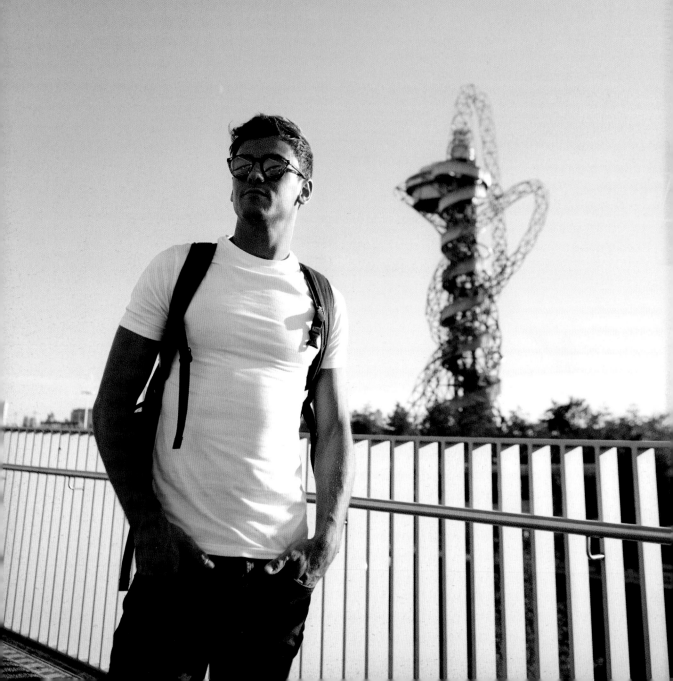

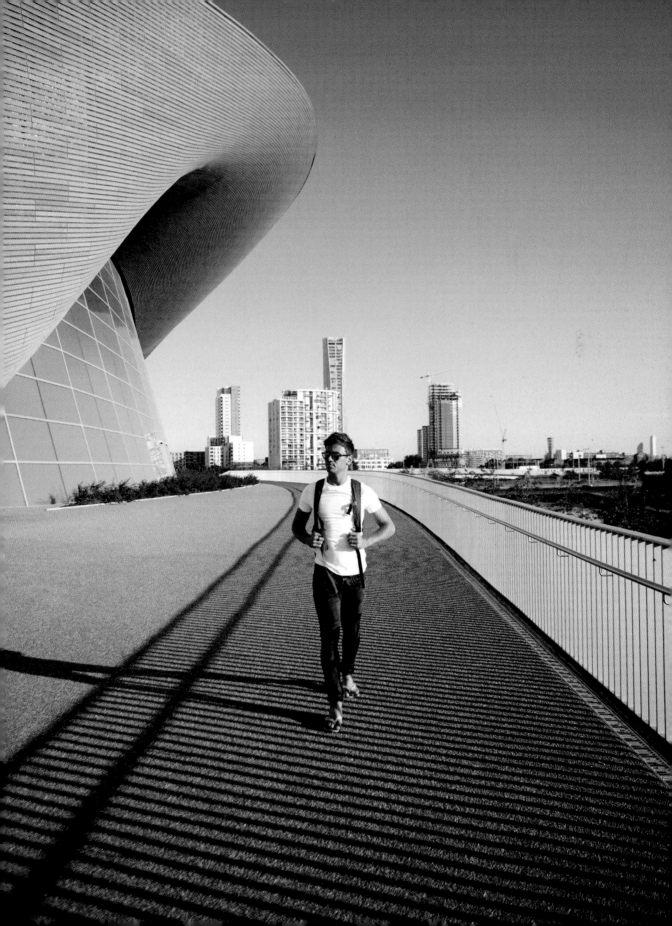

THURSDAY: ARMS AND CARDIO
20-MINUTE ROUTINE

SEQUENCE

**60 SECONDS
JOG/SPRINT**

**30 SECONDS
PRESS-UPS**

**60 SECONDS
JOG/SPRINT**

**30 SECONDS
TRICEPS DIPS**

REPETITIONS

BEGINNERS

Warm up.
Repeat the sequence six times,
resting for 30 seconds to one
minute between each.
Cool down.

INTERMEDIATE

Warm up.
Repeat the sequence twice
Rest for one minute.
Repeat the sequence twice
Rest for one minute.
Repeat the sequence twice
Rest for one minute.
Cool down.

ADVANCED

Warm up.
Repeat the sequence three times
Rest for one minute.
Repeat the sequence three times
Rest for one minute.
Cool down.

ARMS AND CARDIO

HERE'S WHAT TO DO

Start with a warm-up: jog or march on the spot for 30 seconds; follow this with 30 seconds of arm swings, 30 seconds of basic squats, then 30 seconds of shallow lunges. Then follow the routine on the opposite page at the appropriate repetitions level – beginners, intermediate or advanced.

JOG/SPRINT

1 Jog or sprint and as your fitness builds, increase your speed.

2 If you're outside, jog or sprint in laps around the garden or park. If you're at home, jog on the spot.

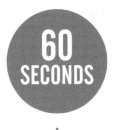

60 SECONDS

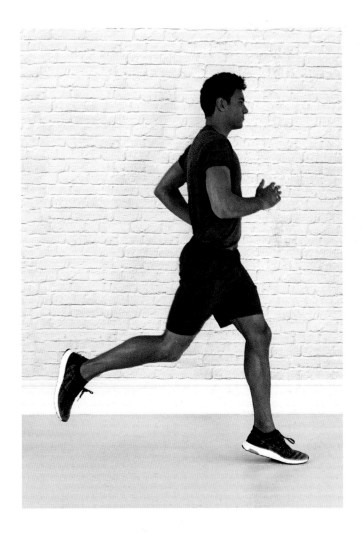

THURSDAY: ARMS AND CARDIO

PRESS-UPS

1 Get into a high plank position with your hands underneath your shoulders. Your arms should be fully extended, your palms flat and fingers facing forwards. Keep your legs straight and knees off the floor.

2 Bend your arms at your elbows, lowering your chest until it is about two inches above the floor and your elbows reach 90 degrees. Keep your back and legs straight at all times. Push back up, trying not to bend or arch your back. Repeat.

EASIER OPTION

Rest your knees on the floor but ensure your core is engaged at all times.

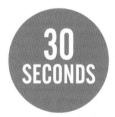

30 SECONDS

REPEAT
60 SECONDS
JOG/SPRINT

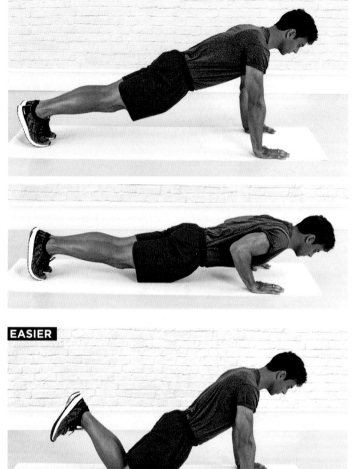

EASIER

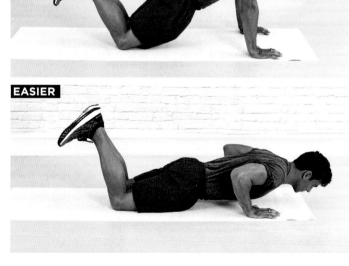

EASIER

ARMS AND CARDIO

TRICEPS DIPS

1 Make sure the chair you are going to use is stable. Position yourself in front of the chair with your knees bent and your hands holding the edge of the chair, fingers pointing towards your body. Keep your back straight and shoulders down. Point your toes up.

2 Bend your elbows to lower your hips towards the floor, again keeping your back straight and your shoulders down. Lift up and repeat.

TO WORK HARDER

Stretch your feet out in front of you and lower your hips as before.

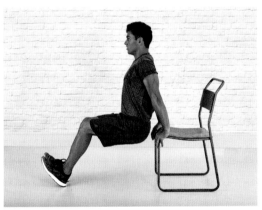

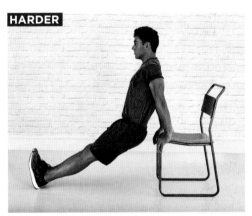
HARDER

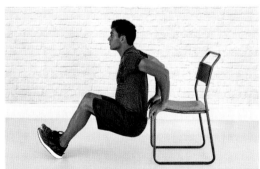

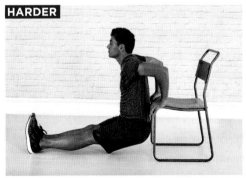
HARDER

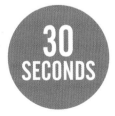
30 SECONDS

THURSDAY: ARMS AND CARDIO

COOL DOWN AND STRETCHES

To cool down, walk for two minutes and regulate your breathing. Then stretch the muscles of whatever part of the body you've been working on. Here are some stretches to do after your arm and cardio routine.

TRICEPS STRETCH

Put your right arm behind your head and reach your hand as far down your back as you can. Grasp your right elbow with your left hand. Pull down and back and hold for 20–30 seconds. Keep your head up. Repeat on the other side.

SHOULDER STRETCH

Bring your right arm across your body. Support it with your left arm and push gently to increase the stretch. Hold for 20–30 seconds. Repeat on the other side.

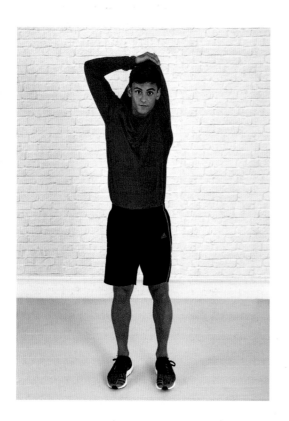
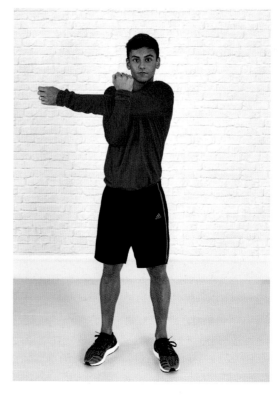

FRIDAY: MORE CORE AND CARDIO
20-MINUTE ROUTINE

SEQUENCE

**60 SECONDS
JUMPING JACKS**

**30 SECONDS
SIT-UPS**

**60 SECONDS
JUMPING JACKS**

**30 SECONDS
PLANK**

REPETITIONS

BEGINNERS

Warm up.
Repeat the sequence six times,
resting for 30 seconds to one
minute between each.
Cool down.

INTERMEDIATE

Warm up.
Repeat the sequence twice
Rest for one minute.
Repeat the sequence twice
Rest for one minute.
Repeat the sequence twice
Rest for one minute.
Cool down.

ADVANCED

Warm up.
Repeat the sequence three times
Rest for one minute.
Repeat the sequence three times
Rest for one minute.
Cool down.

FRIDAY: MORE CORE AND CARDIO

HERE'S WHAT TO DO

Start with a warm-up: jog or march on the spot for 30 seconds; follow this with 30 seconds of arm swings, 30 seconds of basic squats, then 30 seconds of shallow lunges. Then follow the routine on the previous page at the appropriate repetitions level – beginners, intermediate or advanced.

JUMPING JACKS

1 Stand tall with your arms by your sides and your knees slightly bent.

2 Jump up, extending your arms and legs out into a star shape. Land softly, with your knees together and your hands by your sides. Keep your abs tight and your back straight throughout.

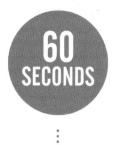

60 SECONDS

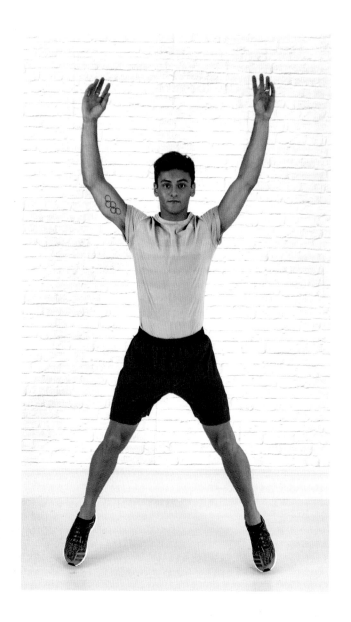

MORE CORE AND CARDIO

SIT-UPS

1 Lie down on your back with your knees bent and your hands behind your ears.

2 Keeping your lower back pressed into the floor, slowly raise your back off the floor. Don't use your hands to pull your neck up, and tuck your neck into your chest as you rise.

3 Come up to a sitting position, then slowly lower yourself down.

TO WORK HARDER

When you're in a sitting position, lift both your legs to a 90-degree angle. Lower them to the floor at the same time as you lower your back to the floor.

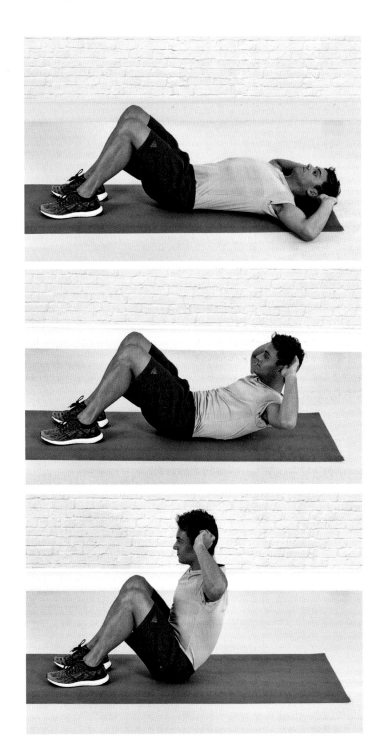

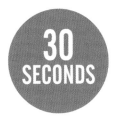

30 SECONDS

REPEAT
60 SECONDS
JUMPING JACKS

FRIDAY: MORE CORE AND CARDIO

PLANK

1 Lie on your front propped up on your forearms and your toes.

2 Keep your legs straight and hips raised to create a straight and rigid line from head to toe. Your shoulders should be directly above your elbows. Keep looking down at the floor.

3 Focus on keeping your abs engaged during the exercise.

EASIER OPTION

Rest your knees on the floor, but ensure your core is engaged at all times.

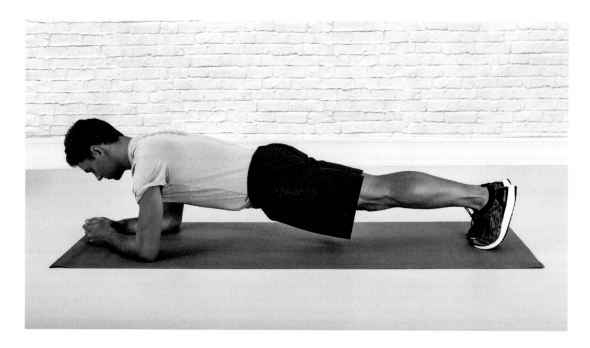

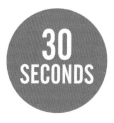

30 SECONDS

MORE CORE AND CARDIO

COOL DOWN AND STRETCHES

To cool down, walk for two minutes and regulate your breathing. Then stretch the muscles of whatever part of the body you've been working on. Here are some stretches to do after your core and cardio routine.

BACK STRETCH

Get down on your hands and knees. Drop your head down and round your back as much as possible – angry cat! Hold for 20–30 seconds.

Then lift your head and arch your back as far as you can – happy cat! Hold for 20–30 seconds, then repeat.

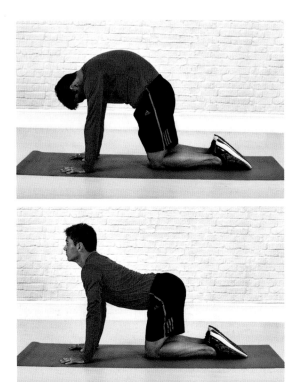

SEAL STRETCH

Lie on your front with your hands under your shoulders. Push up, arching your back and stretching your stomach. Go far enough to feel a good stretch without straining your lower back and hold for 20–30 seconds. Repeat.

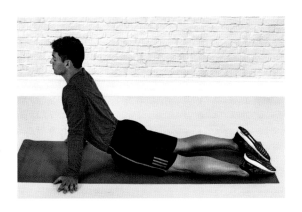

SATURDAY: ALL OVER BODY
20-MINUTE ROUTINE

SEQUENCE

**60 SECONDS
SIDE SHUFFLES**

**30 SECONDS
BURPEES**

**60 SECONDS
SIDE SHUFFLES**

**30 SECONDS
MOUNTAIN CLIMBERS**

REPETITIONS

BEGINNERS

Warm up.
Repeat the sequence six times,
resting for 30 seconds to one
minute between each.
Cool down.

INTERMEDIATE

Warm up.
Repeat the sequence twice
Rest for one minute.
Repeat the sequence twice
Rest for one minute.
Repeat the sequence twice
Rest for one minute.
Cool down.

ADVANCED

Warm up.
Repeat the sequence three times
Rest for one minute.
Repeat the sequence three times
Rest for one minute.
Cool down.

ALL OVER BODY

HERE'S WHAT TO DO

Start with a warm-up: jog or march on the spot for 30 seconds; follow this with 30 seconds of arm swings, 30 seconds of basic squats, then 30 seconds of shallow lunges. Then follow the routine on the opposite page at the appropriate repetitions level – beginners, intermediate or advanced.

SIDE SHUFFLES

1 Adopt a position like a speed skater, leaning forwards slightly. Extend one leg to the side of your body. Extend the arm on the same side and bring the other arm to the front of your body.

2 Jump up and as you come down, extend your arm and leg on the other side.

3 Keep going, switching legs each time.

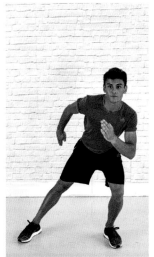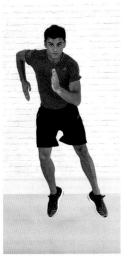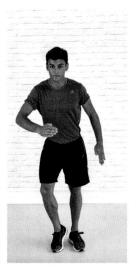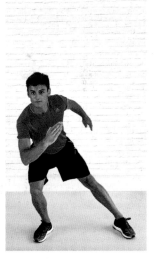

60 SECONDS .....

SATURDAY: ALL OVER BODY

BURPEES

A burpee consists of four separate moves. Start in a standing position.

1 Drop into a squat with your hands flat on the floor.

2 Kick your legs and feet back into a push-up position.

3 Jump your feet forwards again, back into a squat position.

4 Jump up with your arms extending over your head.

EASIER OPTION

Don't kick out into a push-up position and stand up instead of jumping up.

TO WORK HARDER

Lower your chest to the floor when you go into a push-up position.

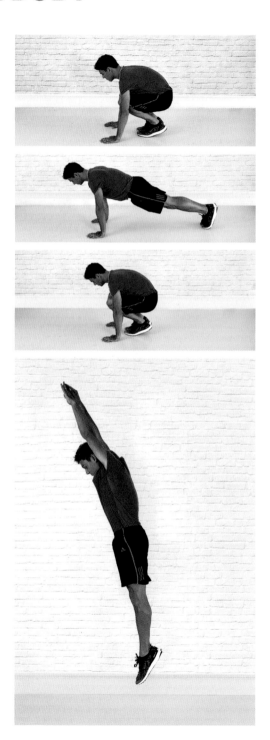

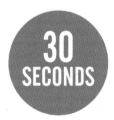

30 SECONDS

REPEAT
60 SECONDS
SIDE SHUFFLES

ALL OVER BODY

MOUNTAIN CLIMBERS

1 Assume a press-up position so your hands are directly under your chest and shoulder width apart. Keep your arms straight.

2 Lift your right foot off the floor and raise your knee as close to your left arm as you can manage.

3 Return to the starting position and repeat with your left leg, raising the knee towards your right arm.

If you are new to this exercise, perform the knee to chest motion slowly at first. Build up your pace with practice.

TO WORK HARDER

Try placing your feet on an elevated platform, such as the bottom step of the stairs. This will make the mountain climbers more difficult.

30 SECONDS

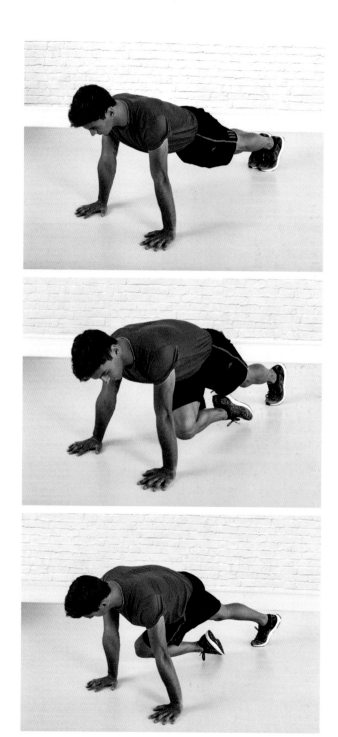

SATURDAY: ALL OVER BODY

COOL DOWN AND STRETCHES

To cool down, walk for two minutes and regulate your breathing. Then stretch the muscles of whatever part of the body you've been working on. Here are some stretches to do after your all over body routine.

CALF STRETCH

Stand with your right leg in front of your left leg. Bend your front leg and lunge forward, keeping the back foot on the ground and the back leg straight, until you feel a stretch. Hold for 20–30 seconds, then repeat on the other side.

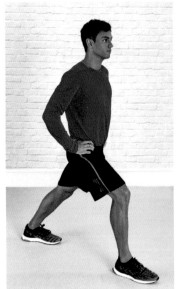 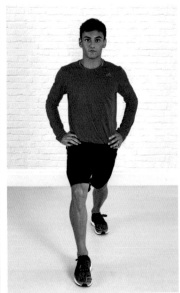

CROSS BODY STRETCH

Lie on your back. Cross your left leg over your body while keeping your shoulders flat on the floor and your arms out at your sides. Keep the leg slightly bent. For a stronger stretch, use your right arm to pull your leg across your body. Hold for 20–30 seconds, then repeat on the other side.

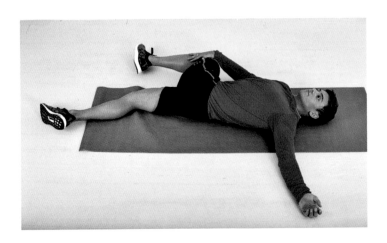

≈ EXTRA STRETCHES ≈

These are great general stretches to do after any routine as part of your cool down.

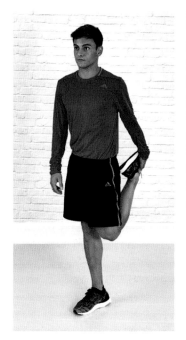

QUAD STRETCH

Stand with your legs together. Bend your left knee back and hold on to your foot to pull the leg back, stretching the front of your thigh. Keep your knees together and your core engaged. Hold for 20–30 seconds, then repeat on the other side.

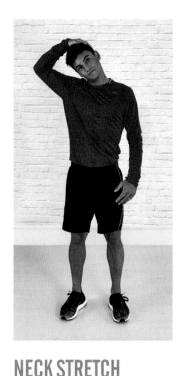

NECK STRETCH

Place your right hand on the side of your head and gently pull your head to one side. Look straight ahead and try to keep your shoulders down. Hold for about 20–30 seconds, then repeat on the other side.

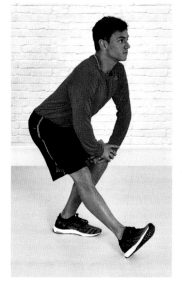

HAMSTRING STRETCH

Stand with your right leg in front of your left. Bend your left knee, while pushing your bum back and your chest up. For a stronger stretch, lift the toes on your right foot. Hold for 20–30 seconds, then repeat on the other side

≈ SUNDAY: REST DAY ≈

You've worked hard all week, so give yourself the day off – you deserve it.
Enjoy a brunch or a Sunday roast and relax, ready to start again on Monday!

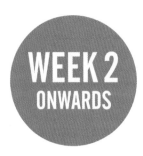

From Week 2 onwards you should start to see an
improvement in your fitness as you do the routines.

As you recover more quickly, move up a level, so if you are a
beginner, go from resting every set to only having one rest
period every two sets and so on.

When the exercises start to feel easier, use the adaptations
to make them harder. For example, do chest-to-floor burpees
or press-ups on your toes rather than your knees.

Stick with it because after a few weeks, you will feel much
fitter, stronger and more energised! Good luck!

NUTRITIONAL INFO

The pages that follow list nutritional details for each recipe, giving the calories and the amount in grams of protein, carbohydrate, sugar, fat, saturated fat, fibre and salt. Note that the sugar content given includes the natural sugars in foods such as milk and fruit as well as free sugars – the sugar added to food. Optional ingredients are not included. Figures below are per serving, unless otherwise specified.

We also list how much each recipe contributes to your recommended vegetable and fruit intake – your '5 a day'. One portion is about 80 grams so in some recipes, there might not be enough veg or fruit in a serving to qualify as a full portion. Five portions of veg and fruit a day is the minimum amount so it's great if you have more!

For someone eating 2,000 calories a day, the suggested level of intake of nutrients is as follows:

Protein (g) 45g

Carbs (g) 270g

Sugar (g) 90g

Fat (g) 70g

Saturated fat (g) 20g

Fibre (g) 30g

Salt (g) 6g

BREAKFAST AND BRUNCH

PLUM YOGHURT POTS/ BANANA/ STRAWBERRY
Page 12
Kcals 265/324/221
Protein (g) 10.4/10/8.5
Carbs (g) 17/23/12.5
Sugar (g) 14.5/19/12
Fat (g) 16/20/15
Sat fat (g) 8/8/8
Fibre (g) 6.5/6/2
Salt (g) 0.2/0.2/0.2
0 of your 5 a day/0/0

BLUEBERRY, BANANA AND SEED PANCAKES (PER PANCAKE)
Page 14
Kcals 97
Protein (g) 4.2
Carbs (g) 9.5
Sugar (g) 8
Fat (g) 4
Sat fat (g) 1.7
Fibre (g) 3
Salt (g) 0.1
0 of your 5 a day

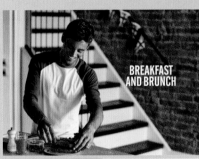

CHEESY RICOTTA AND HERB PANCAKES (PER PANCAKE)
Page 16
Kcals 79
Protein (g) 4.5
Carbs (g) 2
Sugar (g) 0.5
Fat (g) 6
Sat fat (g) 2
Fibre (g) 0.7
Salt (g) 0.1
0 of your 5 a day

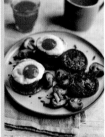
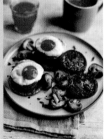

BAKED BREAKFAST MUFFINS WITH CRISPY 'FRIED' BREAD
Page 18
Kcals 527
Protein (g) 31
Carbs (g) 33
Sugar (g) 5
Fat (g) 28
Sat fat (g) 8
Fibre (g) 7
Salt (g) 2.8
1 of your 5 a day

SCRAMBLED EGGS TOM'S WAY
Page 20
Kcals 319
Protein (g) 25
Carbs (g) 1.5
Sugar (g) 1.5
Fat (g) 23
Sat fat (g) 9
Fibre (g) 1
Salt (g) 0.9
1 of your 5 a day

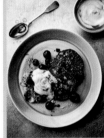
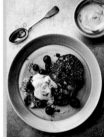

BOILED EGGS WITH SPICED PITTA DIPPERS
Page 21
Kcals 291
Protein (g) 18.5
Carbs (g) 18.5
Sugar (g) 1
Fat (g) 15.5
Sat fat (g) 5.5
Fibre (g) 0.8
Salt (g) 0.9
0 of your 5 a day

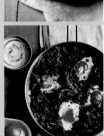

SPINACH AND EGGS
Page 22
Kcals 300
Protein (g) 22
Carbs (g) 6.5
Sugar (g) 3.5
Fat (g) 19
Sat fat (g) 6.5
Fibre (g) 5
Salt (g) 0.8
2 of your 5 a day

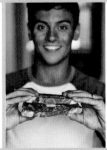

THE ULTIMATE BACON BUTTY
Page 24
Kcals 290
Protein (g) 11
Carbs (g) 23
Sugar (g) 4
Fat (g) 16
Sat fat (g) 3.5
Fibre (g) 4.5
Salt (g) 1.2
2 of your 5 a day

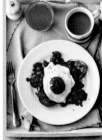

QUICK HOME-MADE BEANS WITH HEALTHY 'FRIED' EGGS
Page 26
Kcals 456
Protein (g) 25
Carbs (g) 48
Sugar (g) 11
Fat (g) 15
Sat fat (g) 6
Fibre (g) 14.5
Salt (g) 1.4
2 of your 5 a day

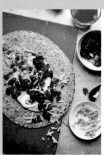

BREAKFAST BURRITOS/EGG/ BACON
Page 29
Kcals 384/404/378
Protein (g) 21/25/18
Carbs (g) 44/43/43
Sugar (g) 6/5/5
Fat (g) 11.5/13.13
Sat fat (g) 5.5/5/5.5
Fibre (g) 9/9/9
Salt (g) 1.6/1.7/1.5
1 of your 5 a day

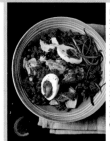

KEDGEREE WITH SALMON
Page 30
Kcals 495
Protein (g) 31
Carbs (g) 33
Sugar (g) 3
Fat (g) 25
Sat fat (g) 5
Fibre (g) x
Salt (g) 0.6
0 of your 5 a day

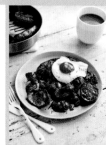

TOM'S BIG FRY-UP
Page 32
Kcals 516
Protein (g) 25.5
Carbs (g) 38
Sugar (g) 13
Fat (g) 27
Sat fat (g) 7.5
Fibre (g) 9
Salt (g) 1.8
2 of your 5 a day

SIMPLE PORRIDGE/FIG TOPPING/MANGO
Page 34
Kcals 400/460/385
Protein (g) 15/15/14
Carbs (g) 45/52/45
Sugar (g) 18/25/18
Fat (g) 17/20/15
Sat fat (g) 6.5/7/9
Fibre (g) 4.5/6/5/6
Salt (g) 0.3/0.3/0.3
0 of your 5 a day

TOAST-IN-THE-PAN GRANOLA
Page 35
Kcals 266
Protein (g) 5
Carbs (g) 22
Sugar (g) 8.5
Fat (g) 12
Sat fat (g) 4
Fibre (g) 3
Salt (g) 0

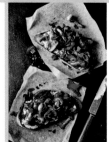

MUSHROOMS ON TOAST
Page 37
Kcals 182
Protein (g) 6.5
Carbs (g) 20
Sugar (g) 2.5
Fat (g) 7
Sat fat (g) 4
Fibre (g) 2.5
Salt (g) 0.5
2 of your 5 a day

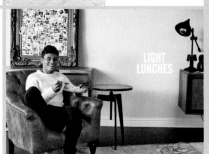

LIGHT LUNCHES

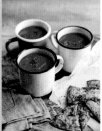

SIMPLE RED LENTIL SOUP WITH CHEESY TORTILLA WEDGES
Page 44
Kcals 300
Protein (g) 15
Carbs (g) 41
Sugar (g) 7
Fat (g) 8
Sat fat (g) 3
Fibre (g) 6
Salt (g) 1.6
1 of your 5 a day

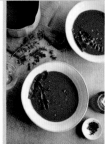

ROASTED SQUASH SOUP
Page 46
Kcals 114
Protein (g) 3
Carbs (g) 13
Sugar (g) 9
Fat (g) 5
Sat fat (g) 1
Fibre (g) 4
Salt (g) 1.2
2 of your 5 a day

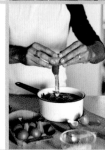

EGG-DROP SOUP
Page 48
Kcals 312
Protein (g) 21
Carbs (g) 8
Sugar (g) 6.5
Fat (g) 20
Sat fat (g) 7
Fibre (g) 9
Salt (g) 2.3
3 of your 5 a day

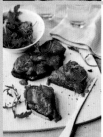

RAREBIT ON RYE
Page 51
Kcals 325
Protein (g) 15
Carbs (g) 20
Sugar (g) 2.5
Fat (g) 20
Sat fat (g) 8
Fibre (g) 4.5
Salt (g) 1.3
1 of your 5 a day

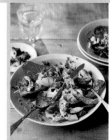

TOM'S CHICKEN CAESAR SALAD
Page 52
Kcals 380
Protein (g) 39
Carbs (g) 9
Sugar (g) 2
Fat (g) 20
Sat fat (g) 5
Fibre (g) 3
Salt (g) 1.1
1 of your 5 a day

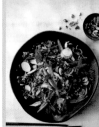

CHICKEN AND MANGO SALAD WITH NOODLES
Page 54
Kcals 426
Protein (g) 33
Carbs (g) 47
Sugar (g) 12
Fat (g) 10
Sat fat (g) 2
Fibre (g) 6
Salt (g) 0.8
1 of your 5 a day

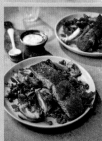

GRILLED SALMON SALAD
Page 56
Kcals 474
Protein (g) 37
Carbs (g) 6.5
Sugar (g) 4
Fat (g) 32
Sat fat (g) 6
Fibre (g) 5
Salt (g) 0.2
2 of your 5 a day

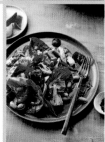

TUNA AND BEAN SALAD
Page 58
Kcals 269
Protein (g) 25
Carbs (g) 14
Sugar (g) 5
Fat (g) 11
Sat fat (g) 1.5
Fibre (g) 6.5
Salt (g) 0.7
2 of your 5 a day

BLACK BEAN STEW
Page 60
Kcals 181
Protein (g) 11
Carbs (g) 22
Sugar (g) 3
Fat (g) 4.5
Sat fat (g) 1
Fibre (g) 5
Salt (g) 1.1
1 of your 5 a day

POACHED EGG SALAD
Page 61
Kcals 307
Protein (g) 14.5
Carbs (g) 27
Sugar (g) 5
Fat (g) 14.5
Sat fat (g) 3
Fibre (g) 5
Salt (g) 0.5
2 of your 5 a day

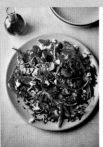

TOM'S SAVOURY FRUIT SALAD
Page 63
Kcals 408
Protein (g) 13
Carbs (g) 19
Sugar (g) 18
Fat (g) 23
Sat fat (g) 9
Fibre (g) 5.5
Salt (g) 1.3
2 of your 5 a day

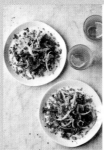

SUMMER SALAD
Page 64
Kcals 268
Protein (g) 8
Carbs (g) 28
Sugar (g) 8
Fat (g) 12.5
Sat fat (g) 1.5
Fibre (g) 7.5
Salt (g) 0.1
2 of your 5 a day

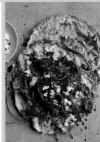

NO-BREAD WRAP/ TUNA FILLING/ ASIAN-STYLE SALAD
Page 66
Kcals 259/251/228
Protein (g) 20/27/25
Carbs (g) 2.5/2.8/8
Sugar (g) 2.5/2.5/7.5
Fat (g) 19/14/14
Sat fat (g) 8/3/3.5
Fibre (g) 0.7/1.5/4
Salt (g) 1.4/0.9/1.1
0 of your 5 a day/0/1

CAULIFLOWER RICE
Page 68
Kcals 52
Protein (g) 1.5
Carbs (g) 4
Sugar (g) 3
Fat (g) 3.5
Sat fat (g) 0.5
Fibre (g) 1
Salt (g) trace
0 of your 5 a day

CAULIFLOWER STEAKS
Page 68
Kcals 26
Protein (g) 1
Carbs (g) 2
Sugar (g) 1
Fat (g) 1.5
Sat fat (g) 0.2
Fibre (g) 0.7
Salt (g) trace
0 of your 5 a day

WHITE BEAN PATTIES
Page 69
Kcals 163
Protein (g) 7.5
Carbs (g) 18
Sugar (g) 1.5
Fat (g) 5
Sat fat (g) 0.5
Fibre (g) 7
Salt (g) 0.2
0 of your 5 a day

HUMMUS
Page 69
Kcals 137
Protein (g) 5.5
Carbs (g) 7.5
Sugar (g) 0
Fat (g) 8
Sat fat (g) 1.5
Fibre (g) 5
Salt (g) trace
0 of your 5 a day

MARINATED FETA
Page 69
Kcals 73
Protein (g) 4
Carbs (g) 0.5
Sugar (g) 0.5
Fat (g) 6.5
Sat fat (g) 3.5
Fibre (g) 0
Salt (g) 0.6
0 of your 5 a day

ROASTED PLUM TOMATOES
Page 69
Kcals 45
Protein (g) 0.6
Carbs (g) 3.5
Sugar (g) 3.5
Fat (g) 3
Sat fat (g) 0.5
Fibre (g) 1
Salt (g) 0
1 of your 5 a day

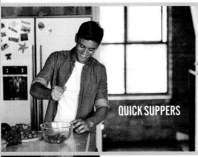

QUICK SUPPERS

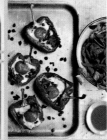

BAKED EGGS IN PEPPERS
Page 76
Kcals 257
Protein (g) 21
Carbs (g) 9
Sugar (g) 8
Fat (g) 14
Sat fat (g) 3.5
Fibre (g) 7
Salt (g) 1.4
3 of your 5 a day

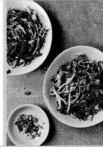

VEGETARIAN PAD THAI
Page 78
Kcals 400
Protein (g) 16
Carbs (g) 67
Sugar (g) 23
Fat (g) 6
Sat fat (g) 2
Fibre (g) 6
Salt (g) 2
2 of your 5 a day

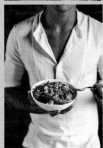

NOODLE SALAD
Page 80
Kcals 596
Protein (g) 40
Carbs (g) 71
Sugar (g) 16
Fat (g) 13
Sat fat (g) 2
Fibre (g) 16
Salt (g) 3.6
4 of your 5 a day

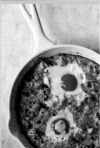

CAULIFLOWER AND EGG HASH BROWNS
Page 82
Kcals 333
Protein (g) 23
Carbs (g) 8
Sugar (g) 6
Fat (g) 22
Sat fat (g) 7
Fibre (g) 3.5
Salt (g) 0.8
2 of your 5 a day

CHILLI-SPICED CHICKPEAS WITH SPINACH AND EGGS
Page 84
Kcals 400
Protein (g) 23
Carbs (g) 19
Sugar (g) 11
Fat (g) 24
Sat fat (g) 5
Fibre (g) 7
Salt (g) 1.5
3 of your 5 a day

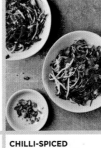

SPICED SQUASH AND BUTTERBEANS
Page 85
Kcals 521
Protein (g) 19
Carbs (g) 73
Sugar (g) 16
Fat (g) 14
Sat fat (g) 7
Fibre (g) 15
Salt (g) 1.2
3 of your 5 a day

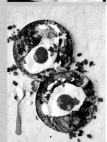

HUEVOS RANCHEROS
Page 87
Kcals 486
Protein (g) 23
Carbs (g) 40
Sugar (g) 7
Fat (g) 24
Sat fat (g) 9
Fibre (g)10x
Salt (g) 1.1
2 of your 5 a day

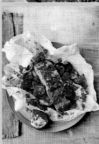

SALMON PARCELS
Page 88
Kcals 485
Protein (g) 35
Carbs (g) 21
Sugar (g) 7
Fat (g) 28
Sat fat (g) 5
Fibre (g) 5
Salt (g) 0.3
2 of your 5 a day

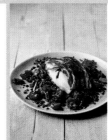

COD AND LENTILS
Page 90
Kcals 343
Protein (g) 37
Carbs (g) 9
Sugar (g) 3
Fat (g) 17
Sat fat (g) 4
Fibre (g) 5
Salt (g) 1.8
1 of your 5 a day

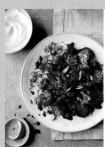

HARISSA PRAWNS
Page 92
Kcals 677
Protein (g) 40
Carbs (g) 49
Sugar (g) 11
Fat (g) 33
Sat fat (g) 4
Fibre (g) 5
Salt (g) 1.2
1 of your 5 a day

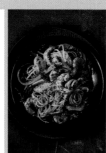

QUICK STIR-FRIED PRAWNS WITH PAK CHOI
Page 94
Kcals 373
Protein (g) 35
Carbs (g) 44
Sugar (g) 2
Fat (g) 6
Sat fat (g) 3
Fibre (g) 3
Salt (g) 1.6
1 of your 5 a day

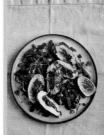

FAJITA-STUFFED CHICKEN
Page 96
Kcals 333
Protein (g) 42
Carbs (g) 15
Sugar (g) 5
Fat (g) 10
Sat fat (g) 3.5
Fibre (g) 6
Salt (g) 0.9
2 of your 5 a day

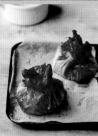

CHICKEN, MOZZARELLA AND PESTO FILO PARCELS
Page 98
Kcals 671
Protein (g) 46
Carbs (g) 43
Sugar (g) 1
Fat (g) 35
Sat fat (g) 16
Fibre (g) 0
Salt (g) 1.6
0 of your 5 a day

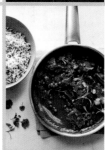

CHICKEN CURRY WITH TOMATO AND COCONUT
Page 100
Kcals 515
Protein (g) 43
Carbs (g) 50
Sugar (g) 8
Fat (g) 14
Sat fat (g) 6
Fibre (g) 6.5
Salt (g) 0.4
2 of your 5 a day

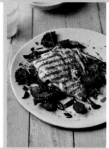

FLAT-IRON CHICKEN WITH BROCCOLI
Page 102
Kcals 300
Protein (g) 43
Carbs (g) 6
Sugar (g) 4
Fat (g) 10
Sat fat (g) 1.5
Fibre (g) 7
Salt (g) 0.5
1 of your 5 a day

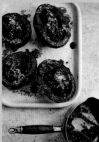

SINGAPORE-STYLE NOODLES WITH PORK
Page 104
Kcals 460
Protein (g) 33
Carbs (g) 53
Sugar (g) 8.5
Fat (g) 11
Sat fat (g) 5
Fibre (g) 8
Salt (g) 0.4
2 of your 5 a day

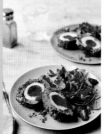

LANCE'S SCOTCH EGGS
Page 106
Kcals 469
Protein (g) 33
Carbs (g) 1
Sugar (g) 1
Fat (g) 37
Sat fat (g) 11.5
Fibre (g) 0.7
Salt (g) 0.5
0 of your 5 a day

GRIDDLED LAMB CHOPS WITH SWEET POTATO MASH
Page 108
Kcals 575
Protein (g) 36
Carbs (g) 27
Sugar (g) 8
Fat (g) 35
Sat fat (g) 19
Fibre (g) 6.5
Salt (g) 1
2 of your 5 a day

VEGETABLE TOTS
Page 109
Kcals 392
Protein (g) 22
Carbs (g) 20
Sugar (g) 2
Fat (g) 24
Sat fat (g) 8
Fibre (g) 4.5
Salt (g) 0.7
0 of your 5 a day

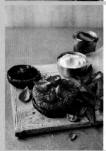

MEATBALL-STUFFED SQUASH WITH SPINACH SAUCE
Page 111
Kcals 500
Protein (g) 43
Carbs (g) 30
Sugar (g) 18
Fat (g) 21
Sat fat (g) 7.5
Fibre (g) 9
Salt (g) 1.7
4 of your 5 a day

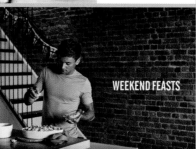

WEEKEND FEASTS

STUFFED SUMMER VEG
Page 118
Kcals 438
Protein (g) 34
Carbs (g) 32
Sugar (g) 18
Fat (g) 17
Sat fat (g) 3.5
Fibre (g) 11
Salt (g) 0.1
5 of your 5 a day

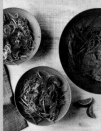

VEGGIE BURGERS
Page 120
Kcals 416
Protein (g) 15
Carbs (g) 64
Sugar (g) 17
Fat (g) 6
Sat fat (g) 1
Fibre (g) 19
Salt (g) 0.6
4 of your 5 a day

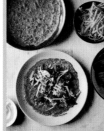

HEALTHY CREPES WITH NO-COOK FILLING
Page 122
Kcals 311
Protein (g) 33
Carbs (g) 21
Sugar (g) 6
Fat (g) 10
Sat fat (g) 3.5
Fibre (g) 1
Salt (g) 2.5
0 of your 5 a day

HEALTHY CREPES WITH 5 MINUTE FILLING
Page 122
Kcals 346
Protein (g) 18
Carbs (g) 21
Sugar (g) 5
Fat (g) 20
Sat fat (g) 9
Fibre (g) 3
Salt (g) 1.3
0 of your 5 a day

HEALTHY CREPES WITH 10-MINUTE FILLING
Page 122
Kcals 487
Protein (g) 35
Carbs (g) 23
Sugar (g) 9
Fat (g) 28
Sat fat (g) 7
Fibre (g) 2
Salt (g) 0.4
0 of your 5 a day

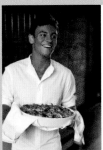

NAN'S BROCCOLI BAKE
Page 124
Kcals 447
Protein (g) 19
Carbs (g) 49
Sugar (g) 6.5
Fat (g) 18
Sat fat (g) 11
Fibre (g) 6
Salt (g) 1.1
1 of your 5 a day

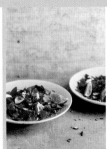

THAI-STYLE CURRY WITH TOFU
Page 127
Kcals 290
Protein (g) 8
Carbs (g) 20
Sugar (g) 9
Fat (g) 19
Sat fat (g) 15
Fibre (g) 5
Salt (g) 2.1
2 of your 5 a day

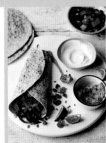

TOM'S FABULOUS FAJITAS
Page 128
Kcals 669
Protein (g) 49
Carbs (g) 62
Sugar (g) 9
Fat (g) 20
Sat fat (g) 4.5
Fibre (g) 19
Salt (g) 1.1
4 of your 5 a day

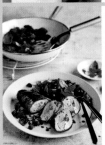

CHICKEN AND BACON PARCELS
Page 130
Kcals 407
Protein (g) 49
Carbs (g) 15
Sugar (g) 5
Fat (g) 15.5
Sat fat (g) 6
Fibre (g) 5
Salt (g) 2
2 of your 5 a day

SWEET CHILLI PRAWNS
Page 132
Kcals 82
Protein (g) 9
Carbs (g) 3
Sugar (g) 3
Fat (g) 4
Sat fat (g) 0.5
Fibre (g) 0
Salt (g) 0.3
0 of your 5 a day

SWEET CHILLI PORK
Page 132
Kcals 106
Protein (g) 11
Carbs (g) 3
Sugar (g) 3
Fat (g) 6
Sat fat (g) 1
Fibre (g) 0
Salt (g) 0.1
0 of your 5 a day

SOY AND GINGER CHICKEN
Page 132
Kcals 84
Protein (g) 12
Carbs (g) 1.5
Sugar (g) 1.5
Fat (g) 3.5
Sat fat (g) 2
Fibre (g) x0
Salt (g) 0.3
0 of your 5 a day

SAUSAGES WITH LEMON AND HONEY DRESSING
Page 133
Kcals 236
Protein (g) 10.5
Carbs (g) 4.5
Sugar (g) 3.5
Fat (g) 20
Sat fat (g) 7
Fibre (g) 0
Salt (g) 0.9
0 of your 5 a day

SIMPLE BEAN SALAD
Page 133
Kcals 138
Protein (g) 7.5
Carbs (g) 12
Sugar (g) 2
Fat (g) 6
Sat fat (g) 1
Fibre (g) 4
Salt (g) 0.2
1 of your 5 a day

THE PERFECT CHOPPED SALAD
Page 133
Kcals 41
Protein (g) 0.5
Carbs (g) 1
Sugar (g) 1
Fat (g) 4
Sat fat (g) 0.5
Fibre (g) 0.8
Salt (g) trace
0 of your 5 a day

CRISPY ASPARAGUS
Page 133
Kcals 29
Protein (g) 1
Carbs (g) 0.8
Sugar (g) 0.8
Fat (g) 2
Sat fat (g) 1.5
Fibre (g) 1
Salt (g) trace
0 of your 5 a day

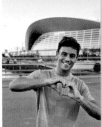

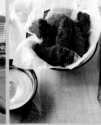

SOUTHERN FRIED CHICKEN WITH WHITE GRAVY
Page 135
Kcals 551
Protein (g) 43
Carbs (g) 32
Sugar (g) 7
Fat (g) 27
Sat fat (g) 10
Fibre (g) 3
Salt (g) 0.9
0 of your 5 a day

MUM'S SUNDAY LUNCH
Pages 136–37
Kcals 753
Protein (g) 60
Carbs (g) 52
Sugar (g) 15
Fat (g) 31
Sat fat (g) 12
Fibre (g) 13
Salt (g) 1
4 of your 5 a day

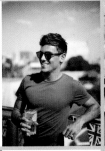

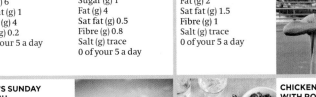

CHICKEN SKEWERS WITH ROASTED VEGETABLES
Page 138
Kcals 603
Protein (g) 50
Carbs (g) 52
Sugar (g) 16
Fat (g) 19
Sat fat (g) 3
Fibre (g) 10
Salt (g) 1.3
2 of your 5 a day

TURKEY MEATBALLS WITH COURGETTI
Page 140
Kcals 300
Protein (g) 39
Carbs (g) 13
Sugar (g) 4
Fat (g) 9
Sat fat (g) 3
Fibre (g) 2.5
Salt (g) 1
2 of your 5 a day

SPICY COTTAGE PIE WITH A MEXICAN TWIST
Page 141
Kcals 518
Protein (g) 31
Carbs (g) 51
Sugar (g) 21
Fat (g) 18
Sat fat (g) 7
Fibre (g) 14
Salt (g) 1.4
5 of your 5 a day

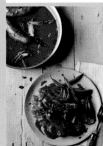

MUM'S SAUSAGE CASSEROLE
Page 142
Kcals 500
Protein (g) 18
Carbs (g) 32
Sugar (g) 20
Fat (g) 31
Sat fat (g) 13
Fibre (g) 10
Salt (g) 1.6
3 of your 5 a day

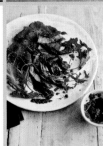

STEAK AND CHIMICHURRI SAUCE
Page 144
Kcals 562
Protein (g) 31
Carbs (g) 32
Sugar (g) 10
Fat (g) 32
Sat fat (g) 7
Fibre (g) 8
Salt (g) 0.6
3 of your 5 a day

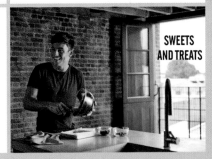

SWEETS AND TREATS

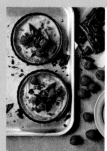

HOT CHEESECAKES WITH A NAUGHTY TOPPING
Page 148
Kcals 474
Protein (g) 10
Carbs (g) 31
Sugar (g) 18
Fat (g) 34
Sat fat (g) 18
Fibre (g) 1.5
Salt (g) 1,1
0 of your 5 a day

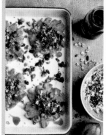

PINEAPPLE CRISP
Page 150
Kcals 300
Protein (g) 6
Carbs (g) 34
Sugar (g) 23
Fat (g) 13
Sat fat (g) 6
Fibre (g) 5
Salt (g) 0
1 of your 5 a day

WHOLEMEAL CHEESY SCONES
Page 152
Kcals 193
Protein (g) 5
Carbs (g) 22
Sugar (g) 1
Fat (g) 9
Sat fat (g) 5
Fibre (g) 1.5
Salt (g) 0.5
0 of your 5 a day

WALNUT DIGESTIVES (PER BISCUIT)
Page 153
Kcals 70
Protein (g) 1
Carbs (g) 6
Sugar (g) 1.5
Fat (g) 4
Sat fat (g) 2
Fibre (g) 0.8
Salt (g) 0.1
0 of your 5 a day

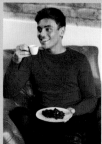

NOT-SO-NAUGHTY CHOCOLATE BROWNIES (PER SQUARE)
Page 155
Kcals 56
Protein (g) 2
Carbs (g) 7
Sugar (g) 6
Fat (g) 2
Sat fat (g) 0.8
Fibre (g) 0.7
Salt (g) 0.1
0 of your 5 a day

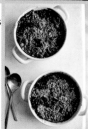

PEAR AND BLACKBERRY CRUMBLE
Page 156
Kcals 256
Protein (g) 3
Carbs (g) 31
Sugar (g) 21
Fat (g) 12
Sat fat (g) 6
Fibre (g) 5
Salt (g) 0.2
0 of your 5 a day

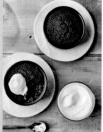

STICKY TOFFEE PUDDING
Page 158
Kcals 346
Protein (g) 7
Carbs (g) 39
Sugar (g) 20
Fat (g) 17
Sat fat (g) 10
Fibre (g) 1.5
Salt (g) 1.2
0 of your 5 a day

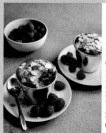

HOT RASPBERRY PUDDINGS
Page 160
Kcals 428
Protein (g) 13
Carbs (g) 38
Sugar (g) 18
Fat (g) 22
Sat fat (g) 3
Fibre (g) 3
Salt (g) 0.6
0 of your 5 a day

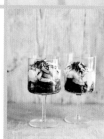

BANOFFEE PIE
Page 162
Kcals 364
Protein (g) 8
Carbs (g) 35
Sugar (g) 24
Fat (g) 20
Sat fat (g) 12
Fibre (g) 4
Salt (g) 0.3
0 of your 5 a day

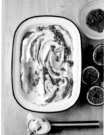

FROZEN YOGHURT/ MANGO AND LIME
Page 164
Kcals 92/113
Protein (g) 5/5
Carbs (g) 13/17
Sugar (g) 12/16
Fat (g) 2.5/2.5
Sat fat (g) 1.5/1.5
Fibre (g) 0/1
Salt (g) 0.2/0.2
0 of your 5 a day/0

CHOCOLATE AND ORANGE FROZEN YOGHURT/ PEANUT BUTTER AND BANANA
Page 164
Kcals 112/148
Protein (g) 5.5/6.5
Carbs (g) 15/16.5
Sugar (g) 14/15
Fat (g) 3/6
Sat fat (g) 2/2.5
Fibre (g) 0.5/0.7
Salt (g) 0.2/0.2
0 of your 5 a day/0

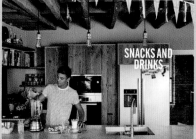

SNACKS AND DRINKS

DATE AND PECAN POWER BALLS /TROPICAL FRUIT (PER BALL)
Page 168
Kcals 47/47
Protein (g) 0.8/1
Carbs (g) 3/5
Sugar (g) 3/4
Fat (g) 3/2
Sat fat (g) 0.3/0.8
Fibre (g) 0.4/1
Salt (g) 0/0
0 of your 5 a day/0

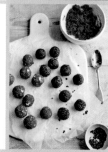

PEANUT BUTTER AND MANGO POWER BALLS/ALMOND AND CHOCOLATE
Page 168
Kcals 37/41
Protein (g) 1/1.5
Carbs (g) 4/2
Sugar (g) 4/2
Fat (g) 1.5/3
Sat fat (g) 0.3/0.3
Fibre (g) 1/0
Salt (g) 0/0
0 of your 5 a day/0

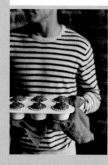

BANANA AND PECAN MUFFINS (PER MUFFIN)
Page 170
Kcals 262
Protein (g) 6
Carbs (g) 32
Sugar (g) 14.5
Fat (g) 11.5
Sat fat (g) 5.5
Fibre (g) 3.5
Salt (g) 0.5
0 of your 5 a day

PEANUT AND COCONUT/ CASHEW/ALMOND (PER 15G TBSP)
Page 172
Kcals 100/90/93
Protein (g) 3.5/3/3.5
Carbs (g) 2/2/1.5
Sugar (g) 1/0.8/0.8
Fat (g) 8.5/7/8
Sat fat (g) 3/1.5/1
Fibre (g) 0.3/0.3/0
Salt (g) 0.1 /0.1/0.1
0 of your 5 a day/0/0

TOM'S CHOCOLATE AND HAZELNUT SPREAD (PER 15G TBSP)
Page 173
Kcals 95
Protein (g) 1.5
Carbs (g) 3.5
Sugar (g) 3.5
Fat (g) 8
Sat fat (g) 1
Fibre (g) 1
Salt (g) 0
0 of your 5 a day

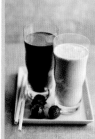

QUICK PROTEIN SHAKE/STRAWBERRY/ CHOCOLATE
Page 174
Kcals 171/181/236
Protein (g) 15/15/17
Carbs (g) 15/17/19
Sugar (g) 13/15/16
Fat (g) 5.5/6/9
Sat fat (g) 1.5/1.5/3
Fibre (g) 1.5/2/4
Salt (g) 0.2/0.5/0.2
0 of your 5 a day/0/0

≈ INDEX ≈

EXERCISES AND LIFE HACKS

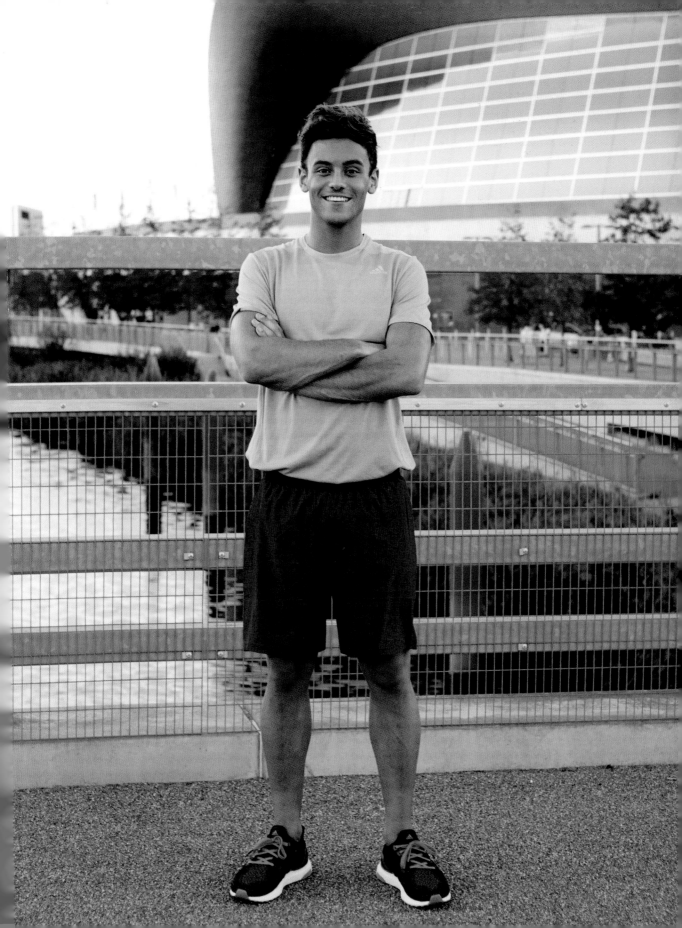

THANK YOU ALL

This book could not have come together without a very special group of people. Huge thanks to the following:

The HQ team, who have shown me such support and brought my book to life: Lisa Milton, Lucy Gilmour, Louise McGrory, Sophie Calder, Alison Lindsay and Nick Bates. I am over the moon with the results!

To Smith and Gilmour for their awesome design work, Dan Jones for his amazing photography, to Emily Jonzen and Morag Farquhar for their perfect styling (my kitchen never looks quite this tidy!), and to Victoria Penrose for make-up and Emily Giffard-Taylor for the clothes for the shoots. To Emma Marsden, who helped me develop and hone my recipes and to Fiona Hunter for her nutritional expertise. Also, to Georgina Rodgers for her enthusiasm and creative input and to my editor Jinny Johnson. What a team!

To my literary agent Rory Scarfe for all his invaluable help and guidance and my manager Tim Edwards, assistant manager Alex McGuire and the rest of the team at James Grant for believing in my passion for all things food and fitness.

To my coach Jane Figueiredo, my strength coach Britt Ducroz and my nutritionist Louise Bloor for helping me learn about what works for my body and how it can help everyone.

To my biggest cheerleaders: Lance for putting up with my endless talk about food and asking when our next meal is; my family for initiating my love for food and the memories that come with it; Sophie, Mike, Sam, Joe and Liam for letting me test my recipes on them and for being so supportive of everything I do. You've all shown me incredible love and guidance through everything in my life.

And last, but by no means least, YOU – thank you for reading my book. I hope you enjoy your Daily Plan.